As America and the healing professions have begun to embrace alternative approaches to health care, children have been left out. This splendid book helps correct this situation. Doctors Ditchek and Greenfield integrate the best of alternative and conventional medicine to help children not only survive but thrive. This is the pediatric medicine of the future because of a simple fact: It works.

—Larry Dossey, M.D., author of *The Extraordinary Healing Power of Ordinary Things* and *Healing Words*

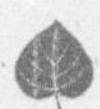

Healthy Child, Whole Child is a groundbreaking synthesis of the best in alternative and allopathic medicine for the very young. Ditchek, Greenfield, and Willeford have written a brilliant and supportive book for all parents. Don't leave the delivery room without it!

—Rachel Naomi Remen, M.D., clinical professor of family and community medicine, University of California at San Francisco, and author of *Kitchen Table Wisdom*

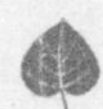

[T]he one book every family should have. Written by two conventionally trained physicians, who also have expertise in alternative medicine, *Healthy Child, Whole Child* lays the foundation for preventing illness and ensuring optimal health for your children. No parent should take chances with the health of a child: thanks to Dr. Stu and Dr. Russ, there is a safe and effective guide that would make Dr. Benjamin Spock proud.

—Kenneth R. Pelletier, Ph.D., M.D., clinical professor of medicine, University of Arizona School of Medicine, and author of *The Best Alternative Medicine: What Works? What Does Not?*

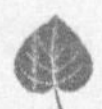

Healthy Child, Whole Child will revolutionize the way children perceive what it means to be healthy. . . . Not only every parent, but every member of our society should own this book and incorporate its message into our lives. Dr. Ditchek, Dr. Greenfield, and Lynn Willeford have defined an innovative and practical model for rearing healthy, whole children.

—Tracy W. Gaudet, M.D., director, Duke Center of Integrative Medicine, Duke University Medical Center

Healthy Child, Whole Child

Healthy Child, Whole Child

Integrating the Best of Conventional and Alternative Medicine to Keep Your Kids Healthy

Stuart H. Ditchek, M.D.

Russell H. Greenfield, M.D.

with Lynn Murray Willeford

Foreword by Andrew Weil, M.D.

wm

WILLIAM MORROW

An Imprint of HarperCollins*Publishers*

Grateful acknowledgment is made to the following:
Published by Clear Light Publishers; Just Imagine, Inc. for permission to reprint material from *Diaphragmatic Breathing* by Rebecca Kajander. Copyright © 1997 by Rebecca Kajander; Guilford Publications for permission to reprint material from *Hypnosis and Hypnotherapy with Children* by Karen Olness and Daniel Kohen. Copyright © 1996 by Karen Olness and Daniel Kohen.

HarperCollins books may be purchased for educational, business, or sales promotional use. For information, please write: Special Markets Department, HarperCollins Publishers, 10 East 53rd Street, New York, NY 10022.

First HarperCollins edition published 2001.

Designed by Jaime Putorti
Line art by Alexis Seabrook

Printed on acid-free paper

The Library of Congress has catalogued the original hardcover edition as follows:
Ditchek, Stuart.
Healthy child, Whole child : Integrating the Best of Conventional and Alternative Medicine to Keep Your Kids Healthy / Stuart Ditchek, Russell Greenfield, with Lynn Murray Willeford.—1st ed.

p. cm.
Includes bibliographical references and index.
ISBN 0-06-273745-7
1. Children—Health and hygiene. 2. Children—Diseases—Alternative treatment. 3. Alternative medicine.
I. Greenfield, Russell. II. Title.
RJ47 .D55 2001
618.92—dc21 00-054113

ISBN 978-0-06-168598-9

11 12 13 OV/RRD 10 9 8 7 6 5 4

To my inspiration, Ruby, and to our children, Teddy, Sammy, Yoni, Batsheva, and Leora. And to my mom and dad, who taught me hope and compassion.

—SHD

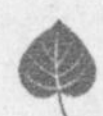

To Julia, our beloved children Abby and Jonathan, my brother Mike, and to our parents of blessed memory—Sophie Greenfield, my source of wonder, and Alexander Greenfield, my hero.

—RHG

To the family and friends who sustain me—you know who you are.

—LMW

This book is designed to give information on various medical conditions, treatments, and procedures for your personal knowledge and to help you be a more informed consumer of medical and health services. It is not intended to be complete or exhaustive, nor is it a substitute for the advice of your child's physician. You should seek medical care promptly for any specific medical condition or problem your child may have. We strongly recommend that you talk to your child's doctor about any measures you use with your child.

All efforts have been made to insure the accuracy of the information contained in this book as of the date published. The authors and the publisher expressly disclaim responsibility for any adverse effects arising from the use or application of the information contained herein.

CONTENTS

SECTION II: therapies

SECTION III: conditions

FOREWORD BY ANDREW WEIL, M.D.

Writing forewords to books is not a high form of the literary art. When I do it, it is usually out of a sense of obligation to author friends or publishers. That is not the case at present. I am genuinely enthusiastic about *Healthy Child, Whole Child,* because it embodies the spirit of the new medicine I have been trying to develop. It is a pleasure to introduce it to readers and to help it find a place in the homes of parents who want to create healthy lifestyles for their children.

I know all three authors of this book, have taught them all, and worked with them. I am proud of their contributions to the growing field of integrative medicine (IM) and delighted that they have taken on the tremendous task of applying it to the realm of children's health.

These are the basic principles of IM:

- A partnership must exist between patient and practitioner in the healing process.
- Good treatment should include appropriate use of all available methods to facilitate the body's innate healing response.
- Physicians must consider all factors that influence health, wellness, and disease, including mind, spirit, and community as well as body.
- Doctors should neither reject conventional medicine nor accept alternative medicine uncritically.

- ▶ Good medicine should be based on good science and open to new paradigms.
- ▶ Doctors should use more natural, less invasive interventions whenever possible.
- ▶ Medicine must address the broader concepts of health promotion and disease prevention as well as the treatment of illness.
- ▶ Practitioners themselves must be models of health and healing, committed to the process of self-exploration and self-development.

Doctors Russell Greenfield and Stuart Ditchek and Lynn Murray Willeford observe all of these principles in *Healthy Child, Whole Child*. I can vouch, especially, for their adherence to the last one, because I know them all to be personally committed in their own lifestyles to health and healing and, as parents, to modeling healthy behavior for their children.

The field of pediatrics is ripe for IM. Pediatricians are open to it. They may lack knowledge and experience of other modalities of treatment because their training failed to provide them, but they have no intellectual barriers in the way of learning. Most parents today want to make use of more natural methods of prevention and treatment for their kids. They are especially wary of using pharmaceutical drugs for all problems. And the healing potential of young people is greater than that of grown-ups. Give their bodies a chance and some support, and they will usually come back to the balance of health quickly, often dramatically.

I have helped produce a textbook for clinicians on Integrative Pediatrics that will be published by Oxford University Press in 2009. The Arizona Center for Integrative Medicine that I direct has trained a number of pediatricians, and we are currently developing a comprehensive IM curriculum (in distributed learning format) that we hope will become a required, accredited component of all pediatric residency programs.

As codirector of the first NIH-funded center for research in alternative medicine in pediatrics, I helped organize studies on the efficacy of cranial osteopathy and echinacea in managing recurrent ear infections and the usefulness of chamomile tea and hypnosis in improving recurrent abdominal pain. Both conditions are very common childhood ailments. A great deal more of this kind of research needs to be done.

But we do not have to wait for the results of studies to come in to apply the basic principles of integrative medicine to raising healthy kids in the twenty-first century. That can be done right away, and Dr. Russ, Dr. D, and Lynn Willeford have done it. I think you will find, as I did, that they have produced a very readable, user-friendly guide that is rooted in common sense and a balanced approach to health and medicine. Raising healthy kids is one of the most important contributions we can make to the future. This book gives you the information and the tools you need to do it.

Tucson, Arizona
April 2008

INTRODUCTION

Are you looking for ways to prevent the umpteen ear infections that kept your daughter on prescription antibiotics most of last year, or at least a better way to treat them? Are you sleep deprived and looking for a cure for your baby's colic? Are you searching for safe, effective therapies to reduce your asthmatic son's reliance on steroid drugs? If you're not concerned about specific illnesses, maybe you have other questions about your child's health. How can I build up his immunity? What will help my child most when she's sick—a drug, an herbal extract, a homeopathic remedy, a chiropractic adjustment, a change in diet, a magnet in her shoe? Can I combine some of these therapies, and how? Which therapies are safe and effective for children and which are useless—or worse, dangerous?

So much has changed so fast in health care that we don't blame parents for feeling out of their depth. Where once there was just one kind of medicine, now there appear to be many, and few parents have the time or the knowledge to sift through and evaluate all the new information on therapies and remedies. More and more drugs are now marketed directly to consumers. The latest medical theories are trumpeted in all the media. Parents are trying to make responsible health care decisions for their children while facing a bewildering array of options and an astounding lack of credible guidance.

At the same time, visits to many conventional pediatricians and family practitioners are getting shorter and less personal. There just isn't time anymore for a physician to delve too deeply into all aspects of a health concern or answer all the questions a family may have. As high technology and concern for the bottom line fray the ties between doctor and patient, medicine spins further away from its roots in a personal healing relationship.

Parents are searching for safer, more natural, more effective, and more caring treatment, instinctively trying to create a system of health care that addresses the mind, body, and spirit in ways that conventional medicine rarely does. Dissatisfaction with a system that doesn't seem to have the time or the inclination to treat a multidimensional individual as well as concerns about the cost and safety of high-tech drugs and therapies have turned many adults toward less conventional health care. Mind/body medicine, homeopathy, herbal remedies, nutritional therapies, acupuncture, massage, body work—a myriad of modalities we never heard of as kids are now widely available new ways of caring for ourselves and our children.

Americans are paying more visits to alternative practitioners than ever before. They're visiting chiropractors for their aching backs, using biofeedback for their headaches, and seeing practitioners of Chinese medicine to relieve the side effects of chemotherapy. They're spending $600 million a year on homeopathic remedies and about $10 billion on nutritional supplements. Medical herbalism, once derided as "folk medicine," is now big business, with major pharmaceutical companies marketing St. John's wort for mood, ginkgo for memory, and echinacea for everything else. And in a lot of cases, hype is outrunning research.

But is this stuff safe for kids? It's one thing to experiment with your own health, but as a parent you have to be more cautious with the health of your children, whose young systems are still developing. Yet with so many conventional and alternative therapies around—some with conflicting philosophies—how can you evaluate them and choose what's best for your children? You need expert help to sort through this information overload, tell you what works and what doesn't, and explain how to combine effective therapies into a well-integrated medical approach.

Consider us your guides through the thicket of pediatric health alternatives now available. We have been well educated and trained in conventional medicine, so we clearly understand its value, yet we are also knowledgeable about the uses of other healing therapies. As practitioners of the "integrative" medicine espoused by Harvard M.D. and best-selling author Andrew Weil, we are trained to draw the best preventive and therapeutic options from a variety of medical systems. Our goal is to advise you on ways to prevent disease and facilitate the optimal functioning of your child's natural healing systems, using the combination of conventional, complementary, and/or alternative therapies that uniquely befit her. This integrative approach respects and works along with other factors in health and wellness, such as nutrition, lifestyle, mind/body interactions, and even spiritual influences. We can give you authoritative, reliable information consistent with medical science, yet we remain open to possibilities beyond our current scientific understanding.

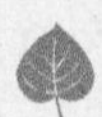

Who are we? Stuart Ditchek (hereafter Dr. D) is a practicing pediatrician and senior founding partner of Integrative Pediatric Associates of New York. Based in Brooklyn, Dr. D's practice carries a caseload of twelve thousand patients, including children who come from great distances to see him. A significant portion of his practice involves high-risk pediatric care and consultation for children and families with serious medical issues. A diplomate of the American Board of Pediatrics, an active fellow of the American Academy of Pediatrics, and a clinical assistant professor of pediatrics at the New York University School of Medicine, Dr. D has all the conventional medical credentials one could wish for in a pediatrician. His style of practice—Integrative Pediatrics—is less conventional, however, drawing as it does on mind/body techniques, botanical remedies, and dietary and lifestyle changes as well as more "accepted" modalities.

In addition to his pediatric practice, Dr. D cares for a diverse group of 240 seriously sick children and teens as medical director at Chai LifeLine Camp Simcha Special, where he has learned to incorporate even more love and humor in his practice. He carries a significant schedule of academic medicine and is a recognized expert in the field of Jewish genetic disorders, advising a variety of organizations and lecturing on this topic and others throughout the United States.

Russell Greenfield (Dr. Russ) is a board-certified specialist in emergency medicine who was one of the first four physician-fellows to train directly with Dr. Andrew Weil in his Program in Integrative Medicine at the University of Arizona. Dr. Russ was the founding medical director of integrative health care for the Carolinas Health Care System and now sees patients in his independent clinical practice. He works with both hospitals and corporations to develop integrative medicine wellness initiatives, and consults with builders and homeowners on the creation of healthy green homes. Dr. Russ travels widely as a speaker, consultant, and instructor on integrative medicine; is a contributing editor to medical books and magazines; and serves as executive editor of an integrative medicine newsletter for health care providers. As an advisor to the Federation of State Medical Boards, he also helped design model guidelines for the practice of integrative medicine.

In addition to being practicing physicians and researchers, we are dedicated husbands and fathers. Dr. D and his wife, Ruby, are raising five children—Leora, Batsheva, Yoni, Teddy, and Sammy—from grammar-school age to college in Brooklyn. Dr. Russ and his wife, Julia, are raising their two school-age kids—Jonathan and Abby—in Charlotte, North Carolina.

We met in 1999 at a seminar put on by the Program in Integrative Medicine at Canyon Ranch Health Resort in Arizona, where Dr. Russ was an instructor and Dr. D was the rumpled attendee whose luggage had been lost by the airlines. While in the gift shop looking for presents for our kids, we began a conversation on the need for a guide to integrative pediatrics for parents. This conversation and friendship has grown and continued over the last ten years as we continue to develop protocols and practices for families to incorporate as integrative approaches.

On the way from casual chat to printed page, we enlisted freelance health writer Lynn Willeford as our partner in this venture. Lynn has the necessary background in integrative medicine, having written for the popular consumer newsletter *Dr. Andrew Weil's Self Healing* since its early days, and having been a research assistant to Dr. Weil on his best seller *Eight Weeks to Optimum Health*. In addition, as the proud mother of a grown son, Lynn is able to provide the long view on raising kids integratively. The book in your hands is, in fact, the one she yearned for two decades ago.

We hope you will read *Healthy Child, Whole Child* from cover to cover, because we believe it is important to have an understanding of the philosophy underlying integrative health care before trying to apply it to your children. In its pages we introduce you to the basic concepts of integrative medicine in general, and integrative pediatrics in particular. We offer the information you need to keep your young children healthy, and advice on what to do when they are not. To stress the importance of optimizing the body's natural healing potential, we've put a discussion of the immune system right in Section I, "Basics," where we also tell you why we think your children should get vaccinations but shouldn't get so many prescriptions for antibiotics. We discuss the behaviors and attitudes that are the foundations of good health: good nutrition, regular exercise, time for relaxation, and protection from environmental and social pollutants. We'll answer such burning questions as: How can I get my kid to eat vegetables? Don't PE classes take care of my child's exercise requirement? Can kids really be stressed? Is it safe to drink the water (or the milk)?

In Section II, "Therapies," we introduce you to other healing approaches that can be included in good pediatric care. You'll learn about osteopathy, massage, botanical medicine, acupuncture, homeopathy, hypnosis, guided imagery, breath work, meditation, biofeedback, energy medicine, and even the power of prayer.

Finally in Section III, "Conditions," we explain when and how these new healing modalities might be useful additions to or replacements for conventional care. We tell how to prevent or treat a sore throat, a cold, an ear infection, a gastrointestinal disorder, asthma, allergies, headache, attention deficit disorder, anxiety, and other conditions common in children. We wrap the book up with resources to help you and your family incorporate healthy behaviors and attitudes into your lives.

There is a clear need for a book like *Healthy Child, Whole Child*. As open-minded conventional physicians with specialized training and experience in complementary and alternative therapies, we felt uniquely qualified to write a guide that honors and supports your child's natural healing potential, tells you what to do now to promote lifelong health for your children, and offers information on safe and effective treatment of common childhood conditions—all from a perspective that values both the art and the science of healing. We hope it will educate and empower you to work with your health care professionals in achieving the goal dearest to our hearts as doctors and parents—wholly healthy kids.

SECTION I

basics

CHAPTER 1

Read This First:

What You Need to Know to Get the Most from This Book

We want to begin by explaining the underlying concepts of integrative medicine. *Integrative medicine* is a term popularized by Dr. Andrew Weil, the groundbreaking Harvard-trained physician and author who founded the Program in Integrative Medicine (PIM) at the University of Arizona. It's a medical model in which:

- The whole person—body, mind, spirit, lifestyle, environment—is taken into account.
- Treatment focuses on the underlying causes of a health problem as well as the symptoms.
- The body's natural capacity for healing is engaged and supported.
- Doctor and patient work in partnership.
- Care is individualized.
- Both conventional and "alternative" therapies are considered.

- Emphasis is placed on prevention of medical problems and promotion of healthy behaviors.

- Gentler therapies with fewer side effects are tried first.

Ideally, integrative medical care promotes well-being by addressing the mind, body, and spirit in a way that is effective, scientifically based, reasonably priced, and free of adverse side effects. With its emphasis on prevention, self-care, and the importance of trying gentle noninvasive therapies first, integrative medicine upsets the whole American paradigm of medicine as a war between doctors and invading diseases. Integrative practitioners work with the whole person—not just a collection of unconnected body parts.

There are many good physicians who are practicing integrative medicine without actually using the term. They are the ones who understand the importance of an ounce of prevention. They really listen to their patients and respect their values. They consider their patients to be partners and are willing to learn about other therapeutic options and discuss them. The very presence of these "mindful doctors" is healing. And yet, our current health care system rewards the practitioners who see the most patients in the least time at the lowest cost. It does not honor those practitioners who take their time and build relationships, which we consider the foundations of good medicine. It is our hope that by partnering with like-minded parents and professionals we can change this paradigm.

Why We Practice Integrative Medicine

Although we are both conventionally trained physicians, the dawning realization that conventional medicine did not have all the answers caused both of us to change the way we practice.

Dr. D's story: I was feeling forced by the constraints of managed care to distance myself from my patients so I could get my work done in the required amount of time. I was losing the passion I had always had for my work because I just couldn't figure out how to treat the presenting problem, discuss preventive strategies for good health, and create the kind of close and caring relationship I wanted to have with my patients and their families in the ten or fifteen minutes that were allocated for a visit.

more on . . .

CONVENTIONAL, ALTERNATIVE, COMPLEMENTARY, AND INTEGRATIVE MEDICINE

Conventional—or *allopathic—medicine* is the mainstream medicine taught in most medical schools and practiced in most hospitals in the industrial world. Its "don't just stand there, do something" attitude makes it excellent for medical and surgical emergencies, but it may be less useful for chronic conditions and unnecessarily aggressive in situations where a little time or a more gentle approach may be equally effective.

Alternative medicine is used separately from or instead of conventional care. It includes therapies or philosophies not generally taught in American medical schools or offered in hospitals in this country. Some, such as Chinese medicine or ayurvedic (Indian) medicine, are considered alternative here, but conventional—or at least traditional—in other countries. After further study or a change in perspective, therapies considered alternative may be incorporated to some degree into conventional medicine. This is what is happening now with mind/body therapies.

Complementary medicine refers to therapies added to conventional treatment but not clinically integrated, so that practitioners may not even be aware of each other's involvement with a particular patient. An example of complementary medicine would be the use of acupuncture, herbal, or nutritional therapies to alleviate the side effects of chemotherapy for cancer without the knowledge or participation of the primary physician. Patients may benefit from complementary treatments, but the term implies an "add-on" to conventional therapy without any significant changes in the core principles of care.

Integrative medicine thoughtfully combines conventional treatment with therapies from both complementary and alternative medicine (CAM). It's more than simply adding more options to the tool bag. We try to create a better environment for healing through a wide range of therapeutic options that address a patient as a whole. We look at possible therapies—conventional and otherwise—with a cautious, scientific attitude, choosing those that are most likely to offer safe and effective treatment for a particular individual.

At the same time, I was also worried that my completely conventional attitude was no longer in sync with patients who were exploring alternative therapies. I was open to ways to avoid the heavy use of antibiotics and high-tech procedures so common in conventional medicine, but I have to admit I wasn't convinced that "herbs and spices" were the way to go.

I decided to research and evaluate these alternatives, in hopes of protecting my patients from adverse side effects or money-hungry charlatans. When I came across the pioneering work of Dr. Andrew Weil, I finally saw a way to increase my focus on preventive medicine, add some safe and effective alternative therapies to my toolbox, and establish a more healing relationship with my patients. Since then I've learned to look more for the root causes of health problems, such as stress or poor diet, and depend less on batteries of tests. My new openness has made the patient-doctor dialogue much more fruitful and has allowed me to relax into enjoying my relationships with my patients. Their parents appreciate this gentle, logical approach toward prevention and treatment that also respects their own insights.

Dr. Russ's story: I loved my work in the Emergency Department (ED), but I was struck by how many of my patients were there because they felt their concerns had gone unheard during their brief visits to their regular doctors. I realized that few of my patients in the ED had any idea how to optimize their health or prevent disease. I also saw an increasing number of patients whose immediate physical problems had been well addressed but whose gaping psychological and emotional wounds had been ignored for so long that they had finally reached a state of emergency. I wanted not only to be able to treat people in the most dire circumstances but also to teach them how to protect their health, so that they might not need the ED. In my free time, I began exploring other approaches to medicine, such as Chinese medicine. In an ideal world, I thought, doctors would be able to use the best, safest, and least invasive therapies from all medical systems to prevent illness and enhance health.

Then one day I came across an article in *LIFE* magazine about the new Program in Integrative Medicine that Dr. Weil was starting at the University of Arizona. I applied for one of the first two-year fellowships at the Program the very next day, and when I was accepted, I quit my job in the Emergency Department and hauled my family from North Carolina to Tucson. At the time I had only a vague idea of what integrative medicine meant, but I hoped it would offer me tools to overcome what I saw as the limitations of conventional medicine.

Naively, I thought I was just making a professional transition; I had no idea that it would require a personal transformation as well. My skeptical mind was frequently forced to acknowledge that conventional medicine had a lot to learn about harnessing our own natural powers of healing. My training at PIM (and the birth of our children) also taught me that children, with their inherently strong healing systems, could benefit greatly from an integrative approach to health.

Dr. Weil's goal was to train agents of change in hospitals, medical schools, government, and the marketplace. Since completing my fellowship, I've been fortunate to direct an integrative medicine center owned and operated by a large health care system, help develop a supermarket chain's wellness initiative, and consult on the building of homes that are not only green but healthy. I believe the necessary changes in medicine and in our society will come even more quickly if we all work together to promote wellness in our schools, in the workplace, and in the home, so that the next generation is healthier than our own and the health care system of our children's children is truly focused on health and healing.

The Principles of Integrative Pediatric Medicine

Integrative pediatric medicine has nine basic principles in common with integrative medicine, as well as one additional principle specific to the care of children. The principles are:

1. *A belief in the innate healing power of the body*. The conventional medical approach is often to ignore or try to override the natural defensive functions of the body by suppressing symptoms. Integrative medicine is more focused on using the best therapies to strengthen and enhance the functioning of your innate healing capability. This principle is especially important in treating children, who have the potential to heal so much faster than adults. As most parents have witnessed, a child can bounce back from a fever or heal a cut virtually overnight.

2. *Recognition of the interaction among body, mind, spirit, family, community, and environment*. The time-pressed conventional doctor generally focuses on what is called "the presenting problem," the symptom that brought

you to his or her office that day. Yet no health problem exists in isolation. Health and illness are often manifestations of the balance—or lack thereof—between all the pieces of our lives.

An integrative practitioner knows the importance of not just looking at symptoms but also listening for deeper issues that might be contributing to the illness. We try to build a relationship with our patient that allows us to know the whole person—not just the medical and family history—but how the patient eats, exercises, sleeps, and relates to his or her environment. We want to know what stressors are present and how the child's body reacts to them.

3. *A conviction that it is better to prevent disease now than treat it later.* Many conventional providers are not as well versed in preventive care because most medical schools have focused on treatment at the expense of prevention. There are now innumerable studies showing the health-protective effects of good food, plenty of water, regular exercise, and reduction of stress, so integrative practitioners make a point of explaining to both patients and parents lifestyle measures to promote health and prevent disease. Educating parents and kids early in such healthy habits as eating well and staying active is a good way to avoid having to treat the same children for type-2 diabetes at age twelve.

4. *The belief that treatment should be customized to individuals.* People vary in so many ways—genetics, medical history, biochemistry, digestion, hormone levels, attitudes, habits, values, environment, weight, age, and gender—that medicine simply cannot be one-size-fits-all. Each of these factors can influence what works and what doesn't in a specific individual. For instance, the same condition may have different causes in different people, so finding the most effective treatment may mean looking at a range of options. Pharmaceutical drugs can vary in their effects four- to fortyfold, so it is especially important to tailor the dose to the individual rather than vice versa. An integrative doctor strives to use the lowest possible dosage that is adequate to the job, recognizing that the effective dose of a prescription drug may well be less than the manufacturer's suggested dosage.

5. *A preference for gentle and inexpensive therapies over invasive or expensive ones.* In most cases we start gently and become more aggressive as necessary. We have seen too many poor outcomes from overintervention, unnecessary drugs, and invasive procedures. For us, in nonemergency situations the first choice for therapy is not the "big guns" but the "small sticks." Why start steroid drug treatment for asthma before seeing if HEPA filters in the home will do the trick? Why surgically insert pediatric ear tubes if a change in diet might produce the same results?

6. *A desire to integrate the best of conventional and "unconventional" medicine.* An integrative practitioner employs a wide-ranging set of tools—from conventional ones such as vaccines, antibiotics, pain medications, diagnostic tests, and surgery to mind/body techniques, nutritional interventions, acupuncture, massage, yoga, botanicals, and other alternatives. We don't turn our backs on the wondrous technological advances of the past few decades. Rather we embrace them, understand their limitations, and build on them.

You have to know when to use what. There are times when only a prescription drug or invasive procedure will do, but there are just as clearly conditions for which conventional medicine has few or no effective options to offer. For instance, we have few satisfactory conventional treatments for viral illnesses, autoimmune disorders, and many forms of chronic headache or pain. In such cases alternative treatments might offer benefit.

Yet alternative therapies range from the well researched to the harebrained. We worry about the millions of Americans who are spending billions of dollars each year on "unconventional" medical, herbal, and dietary therapies without ever telling their primary care doctors what they're doing, leaving themselves unprotected from harmful or ineffective therapies and at risk for adverse interactions between otherwise useful therapies and conventional medications. People need someone with the scientific training to help them evaluate these options intelligently—not the teenager in the health food store, not the Web site with a financial stake in the information it presents, and not the uninformed host of a talk show. You need a physician willing to talk with you about these options in an open and nonjudgmental way.

7. *A determination to forge a healing partnership with patients and parents.* Traditionally, the doctor has always known best, and patients who asked too many questions were treated as if they were challenging the doctor's credentials. Yet more healing actually goes on when the doctor and patient form a partnership in which the patient feels listened to and heard and is accorded the right to participate in decisions about his or her own health. We believe our role as doctors is to offer our findings and judgment and be the patient's knowledgeable guide and advocate. We believe that the relationship people have with their child's pediatrician is the most critical and long-lasting relationship they will have as parents.

An integrative doctor—like any good doctor—knows that better results come not just from understanding the illness but also from understanding the person who *has* the illness. Everyone who comes into our offices has underlying fears that may remain unspoken but need to be discerned and addressed. We encourage our patients and their parents to discuss these concerns. To find out how they perceive their illness and what treatment expectations they have, we listen actively and with empathy. We try to be aware of subtle cues, leave room for any information to be offered that may require courage, and make sure that the parent and patient clearly understand what is to be done and why so they can "buy into" the program. We acknowledge that in health care partnerships patients have the right to make the final decision, although they may choose to cede it to the doctor.

Of course, the concept of partnership implies equal responsibilities too. Along with the right to be an active and welcome participant in health care for your children, you must be willing to exert yourself on their behalf. This may mean searching the library or the Internet for useful information to bring to your child's doctor or changing your own unhealthy behaviors (Big Macs for lunch, too much TV, etc.) in order to be a better role model. It means taking the trouble to find a practitioner who meets your values and connects with and respects your child. Ideally it also means building a partnership with your child that is based on love and encouragement.

It is also important for parents to allow children to accept responsibility for their own health from an early age. Parents cannot fix everything.

Often the key to ongoing issues like headaches or bed-wetting lies with the child.

8. *An acknowledgment that patients and parents have good instincts about their health*. An integrative physician expects to involve patients and their parents in the diagnosis and treatment of their problems. We almost always ask both parents and children what they think the cause or cure for their problem is, and we often find their instincts are right on target. By acknowledging their deeper knowledge of themselves or their children, we empower our patients and their parents. Only they may know the deeper reasons for their condition. We have learned from experience that a stress-related disease is not going to go away for good until the child recognizes its cause, thus starting a process of self-awareness, empowerment, and cure.

We also rely on the fact that most parents have a strong and pure instinct for their children's health and well-being. Parents know whether their baby's cries are from hunger or pain or fatigue, whether they mean "get this wet diaper off me," or "I'm lonely, where is everyone?" They know if something's "off," and most of them have a true sense of when a real problem exists with their child. An "instinctive pediatrician" listens closely to parents and children, staying alert to the verbal and nonverbal cues that transmit this parental sense. It could be a persistent fever that just doesn't seem like other fevers the child has had, a cough or a cry that sounds different, a lack of energy in a kid who is usually running on all cylinders all day long. An observant parent makes a health practitioner's job that much easier.

There is also an additional principle that applies specifically to integrative pediatrics:

9. *The realization that children are not small adults.* When caring for a child we can never forget that we are caring for a complex, developing system and must look at not just the short-term effects of a treatment but its long-term effects as well. We want to be cautious of any therapy that might interfere with the complicated processes that lead to growth and maturity. We must remember that drugs and herbal remedies that are appropriate for adults may not be equally safe for children. Nor does Food and Drug

Administration approval mean that a drug is necessarily safe for all ages and all conditions. The FDA now requires age-specific safety profiles for all new drugs, but a majority of existing pharmaceutical drugs prescribed for children have not actually been approved for pediatric use because they have never been tested to determine the best delivery method, dosage, and duration of therapy for children. Most complementary and alternative therapies have not been tested on children either, a problem that still needs to be addressed.

As integrative practitioners, we also take the emotional effects of any medical procedure into account, especially with children. For example, even the simple, painless echocardiogram seems to upset children to the point that specialists ask us to prescribe sedatives to children undergoing this procedure. CT scan and MRI machines can be particularly scary, so we may use mind/body techniques, music, or aromatherapy to dispel children's fears. Children are also more easily traumatized by a bad experience, which colors how they react if the procedure must be repeated later. Parents can help by maintaining their own calm during necessary procedures.

Consulting an Integrative Physician

What can you expect from an integrative practitioner? In three words—a healing relationship. Integrative pediatricians or primary care providers should be well versed in conventional medicine and be knowledgeable or at least interested in learning about other therapies as well. They will offer advice regarding prevention of disease and optimization of health to all their patients. They will, when appropriate, offer inexpensive, gentle therapies that support the body's natural healing process as a first resort to those who are sick. They may refer to trusted practitioners of other therapies, such as acupuncture, counseling, or biofeedback. Anything will be considered that may safely help the child. Mutual respect between provider, patient, and parent is a priority, so questions about or discussions of therapy are not only welcomed but also encouraged.

Remember, your child's doctor may already provide such caring, informed, and empowering care, without using the label *integrative*. We don't want to suggest that even completely conventional doctors cannot have caring relationships with their patients, because they clearly do. But there is a difference in perspective. An integrative doctor is more likely to provide preventive care or put greater emphasis on supporting the natural process of healing than suppressing symptoms.

Making Any Visit Integrative

If you cannot find a health professional who practices integrative medicine where you live, you can still get health care more in line with your values from a conventional physician or even a health maintenance organization. Parents willing to push for more integrative care for their children have the potential to be a driving force in changing the way medicine is taught and practiced in this country.

- *Keep your own medical file for each family member*. Include doctor visits, test results, medications taken, side effects, and outcome, as well as any supplements taken for the condition or other alternative therapy. Bring your child's file with you to doctor appointments. If you belong to an HMO, your primary care physician may change often, so you need to be familiar with your child's health history yourself.

- *Write down the questions you want to ask*. Then hand the list to the doctor at the beginning of any visit. Take notes when the doctor responds.

- *Don't be afraid to talk to your doctor*. Tell him or her about your health care needs and values—and about your expectations for the doctor-patient relationship.

- *Be honest about all nontraditional approaches that have been tried and whether they worked for your child*. This is both educational for the physician and protective for your child, reducing the risk of drug/herb interactions, for example.

- *If a drug is prescribed, ask if it is needed right away*. Often a "tincture of time" or a few lifestyle changes can do the job just as well. Ask why this particular drug is being prescribed. Has it been tested for safety in children? Is it proven better than the older drug you know works in your child? Is there a similarly effective drug with fewer side effects or lower cost?

▶ *Ask for handouts or other printed materials available on subjects of interest to you.* Ask if there are support or patient-education groups pertinent to your child's problem.

▶ *Educate yourself.* You may need to be the one to find a qualified acupuncturist or a biofeedback trainer. Learn a little about your child's condition from reliable sources. Send copies of pertinent studies or articles to the doctor before the next appointment, with a request for some feedback.

▶ *Be prepared to change physicians if yours is not willing to be open-minded and work in partnership with you.*

TIP: The best way to find a physician who practices integratively is to ask friends for recommendations or ask respected alternative practitioners which M.D.'s and D.O.'s refer patients to them. You can also go online to either the Program in Integrative Medicine at the University of Arizona or the Consortium of Academic Health Centers for Integrative Medicine (see Resources) and search for an individual physician or clinic in your area.

CHAPTER 2

Your Child's Invisible Shield:

Immunity and How to Optimize It

In the days before AIDS and chemotherapy, the average person rarely talked about immunity. Oh, you might say you got a cold because you were run-down or that you needed to build yourself back up after a bout of flu, but there was no general awareness of the role and mechanisms of the immune system. We weren't as fluent in T-cell counts and natural-killer cells as we are today. But since AIDS taught all of us about the importance of a functioning immune system, parents now wonder whether they need to buy products that promise to boost immunity or create "super-immunity" in their kids. So let's talk about immunity—what it is, whether you can improve it, and whether it really needs to be super to do the job.

What Are the Parts of the Immune System?

The immune system is everywhere in the body. It includes specific glands, yes, but also the tiny hairs that line the tubes in your lungs, the mucous linings of your mouth and your gut, the physical and chemical barriers on your skin, the acid in your stomach, and the protective enzymes in your tears and saliva, as well as the cells in your blood and your lymph (the clear fluid that transports immune cells and carries out debris).

The organs of the immune system include the skin, spleen, thymus, bone marrow, lymphatic system, tonsils and adenoids, appendix, and small intestine. Each of them plays a role in the production, storage, or transportation of the multitude of protective cells that are working round the clock to keep infection, chronic inflammation, or cancer from gaining a foothold in our bodies.

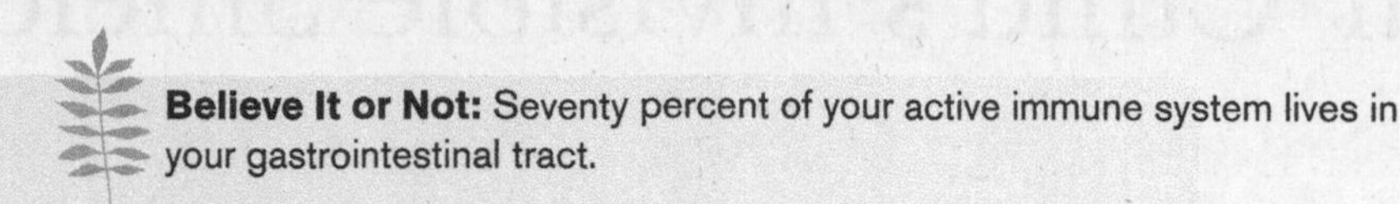

Believe It or Not: Seventy percent of your active immune system lives in your gastrointestinal tract.

Conventional doctors generally view the immune system as a collection of individual organs, each of which has a specialized role to play in maintaining health. Integrative practitioners, on the other hand, tend to look at the entire system as a whole. A properly functioning immune system isn't working only on the skin or in the lymph nodes. It's working all at once in an exquisitely coordinated and well-balanced dance of partners spread far and wide throughout the body.

The members of this defensive system coordinate their activities and communicate back and forth with the brain, endocrine glands, and gastrointestinal tract by way of chemical messengers such as hormones, cytokines, histamine, and neurotransmitters. This intricate machinery (the ultimate in interactivity!) works to maintain that divine balance we call good health.

Good health does not require super-immunity, and we're not sure that products that claim to provide it can actually deliver. All you and your kids need is for the immune systems you were born with to function the way they are supposed to function.

A robust immune system protects you not just from immediate illness but from long-term disease as well. For instance, abnormal cells arise spontaneously in the body all the time, only to be repaired or destroyed by the immune system before they can lead to cancer. Your personal defense system is able to detect and eliminate many chemical carcinogens and natural toxins that enter the body through the air you breathe or the food you eat and repair any damage they have caused. A strong defense against disease-causing agents (pathogens) becomes even more important now that research is suggesting a connection between bacteria and viruses and such long-term conditions as heart disease, stomach ulcers, and some cancers.

What Exactly Does the Immune System Do?

While everyone talks about "building immunity," few understand what's really involved in the day-to-day workings of the immune system. Our bodies are constantly exposed to potentially harmful bacteria, viruses, fungi, parasites, allergens, toxins, pollutants, pesticides, carcinogens, and radiation (even sunlight has its dark side). In fact, we are exposed to so many potential sources of illness that it's a wonder we're not sick all the time! Fortunately, our immune systems are always on the job, repelling invaders, silently erasing cuts and bruises, and restoring regular function to the body after illness.

The primary function of this intricate and infinitely responsive system is to monitor activities throughout the body and protect the body from harmful alien substances. Through experience, the immune system eventually becomes exquisitely sensitive to what is "me" and what is "not-me" and is able to target these foreign substances and either neutralize or destroy them before they can do harm. Sometimes the immune system does this job too well. In autoimmune disorders, immune cells attack the body's own tissues as if they were invaders. With allergies and hypersensitivities, the system responds overzealously to seemingly harmless substances like cat dander or peanuts.

We are rarely aware of the immune system when it is working efficiently. However, sometimes poor diet, stress, lack of exercise, environmental pollutants, or other causes weaken the immune system and allow infectious or inflammatory processes to set up shop. Oddly enough, the symptoms that make you think that your child is sick, like fever or swollen glands, are actually signs that his immune system is mounting a good response. A slight rise in body temperature slows the growth of invading organisms and speeds up immune response, while the swelling of the "glands" (actually lymph nodes) indicates that activated immune cells are gathering there to filter out and neutralize invaders.

more on . . .

NATURAL IMMUNITY

We are all born with individual susceptibilities or resistance to disease that affect the operation of our immune systems. As a species we have protection against some diseases; we don't get feline (cat) leukemia, for instance. Then some of us are more or less susceptible to diseases or conditions by reason of our ethnic or racial heritage. Africans, for example, have greater genetic resistance to malaria than Northern Europeans.

Other forms of immunity are acquired either actively or passively, built up through natural exposure to various pathogens, through vaccinations, and even through your mother's milk, if a child is breast-fed.

How Do Our Immune Systems Develop?

We are born with some innate immune factors (see box above), but the immune system generally learns as it goes along. Babies are born with the "hardware" of an immune system in place: the organs, systems, and the immature cells (called *stem cells*) that will become immune cells. But they must develop their own "software" by teaching the components of the system how to work together. At first a baby operates with the antibodies transferred through the mother's bloodstream while the baby is in the womb and through the breast milk after birth. During birth, some microorganisms from the mother's vagina and perineum get into the baby's mouth. (Children born by caesarean section pick up their first bacteria from the hospital and staff, instead.) These supply the "starter" bacteria for the infant's intestinal tract, where they help digest food, fight harmful bacteria, stimulate the immune system, and even produce vitamins.

The immunity borrowed from the mother wears off in a few months. Because the infant's own immune system has only just begun to develop, this is the time when your child is most vulnerable to serious infection. The immune system will slowly gain in strength as each encounter with a mild and otherwise unnoticed microorganism teaches the developing system how to recognize and deal with these not-me particles. With experience, the immune system becomes more and more skilled at defense and accumulates more memory cells that can quickly produce antibodies. Memory cells from these encounters continue to circulate throughout the body, so the system can jump immediately into a correct response the next time that particular virus or bacteria appears.

The immune system also has to learn which not-me bacteria are actually beneficial, so that it doesn't destroy "good bugs" such as the lactobacilli and bifidobacteria normally found in the digestive tract. All children carry both "good bugs" and "bad bugs" (pathogens) in and on their bodies. The pathogens cause no harm as long as they are kept in place and in balance with other microorganisms. For example, the bacterium *Clostridium difficile* normally lives in the colon, where it is kept in check by the rest of the organisms that compose normal intestinal flora. However, antibiotics may reduce the number of protective bacteria, upsetting the balance and allowing *C. difficile* to reproduce enough to cause an infection.

Young children need exposure to mild pathogens in order to become immune competent. That's why we don't recommend filling children's rooms with antibacterial toys, soaps, bedding, and sprays in an effort to protect them from all contact with germs. Some medical researchers even theorize that this obsession with providing a germ-free environment may backfire over the long term, making children more vulnerable to developing allergies and asthma.

more on . . .

THE "HYGIENE HYPOTHESIS"

Advocates of the "hygiene hypothesis" believe that a germ-free environment deprives very young children of the exposure to innocuous bacteria that is necessary to balance the two arms of the developing immune system. The stronger arm at birth, Th2, drives allergic responses. Th1, the other arm of the immune system, fights infection. Exposure to otherwise harmless microbes typically builds up the Th1 response, equalizing the immune system. However, some say that Th1 responses are not getting a chance to develop and strengthen as they should because so many young children are exposed to antibiotic drugs and antimicrobial products that wipe out all the germs in their inner and outer environments. According to this hypothesis, the increased imbalance in the two arms of the immune system is driving the increase in allergies and asthma that we are seeing today. If this proves to be the case, it might be better to let your children get a little dirty now and then.

Influences on Immunity

Your environment, what you eat, how much you drink, how long you sleep, and how much or how little you exercise all influence the quality of your immune response. Your brain also has tremendous influence on health and healing. There is, in fact, a whole field of study called psychoneuroimmunology that looks at the connections between the brain and the endocrine and immune systems and at how our thoughts and feelings affect the immune system's responses. Research in this field increasingly links factors such as stress and emotions to our susceptibility and response to infections, pain, autoimmune disorders, heart disease, and cancer. One day we will probably take for granted the now-controversial idea that every major organ system and regulatory mechanism in the body is affected by outside events and their interpretation by the mind and emotions.

As evidence for the integration of these systems, researchers point to the fact that the immune system's white blood cells have receptors for chemical messengers from both the endocrine glands and the brain. This chemical communication between the brain, the endocrine system, and the immune system seems to go in all directions—from the brain to the immune system, from the glands to the immune system, from the immune system to the brain, and so on.

Sixteen Ways to Optimize Your Child's Immunity

You can consider the sixteen steps that follow to be your blueprint for raising a healthy child. We will discuss each of them in greater detail in the chapters that follow. Please don't be intimidated by the length of this list. Just start with those steps that seem most achievable for your family and add new ones as you can.

1. *Make sure your children get enough sleep.* Lack of sleep puts significant stress on the body. Haven't you noticed that you get more colds when you've been sleeping poorly? (See chapter 23.)

2. *Feed your kids a balanced, nutritious diet.* Breast-feed your babies for at least a year, or as long as possible, and give older kids lots of fruits, vege-

tables, and whole grains. Minimize the amount of highly processed foods they eat. (See chapter 5.)

3. *Protect your children from environmental pollutants.* Insure that their drinking water is pure. Wash your produce and buy organic foods when possible. Look for foods wrapped in nontoxic materials. Avoid the use of harmful household, lawn, and garden chemicals. (See chapter 8.)

4. *Teach your children how to reduce stress and how to cope with life's inevitable irritations in a healthy way.* As they get older, teach them to stay alert for the origins of some of their health problems in stress, anxiety, or other emotional states. Try to keep your own stress levels in check, as your kids will pick up on your anxieties. (See chapter 7.)

5. *Emphasize basic hygiene.* Teach your kids the proper way to wash their hands and brush their teeth. Hand washing is the first-line protective strategy against colds, flu, and other infections.

6. *Make physical activity a family goal.* Take frequent walks and bike rides together, or play hoops in the driveway after dinner. Limit sedentary activities, such as watching TV or playing video games. Exercise regularly yourself, and tell your children why you do. (See chapter 6.)

7. *Make sure your children drink plenty of water.* This will keep their organs functioning properly and their mucous membranes fat and happy. The mucous membranes that line your body passages are your prime defense against colds, flu, sinusitis, airborne toxins, and even urinary tract infections.

8. *Have fun.* Good times and strong social ties reduce levels of stress hormones and improve immunity. And a sense of humor will get you and your children through many trying times.

9. *Encourage optimism and the desire to be of use in the world.* It's never too early to instill a sense of meaning or spirituality in your children's lives so they feel part of something greater than themselves. Studies have linked positive attitude to faster healing.

10. *Give your children massages and teach them how to massage themselves and other family members.* We all yearn for some form of touch, and loving touch is a great stress reducer. (See chapter 11.)

11. *Get the recommended shots.* Immunization protects our children from diseases that once caused a great deal of pain and suffering. (See chapter 3.)

12. *Avoid unneeded antibiotics and antibacterial products.* The immune systems of your little ones need exposure to the common germs of everyday life to be able to fend off future infections. Recognize that antibiotics do have their place, however.

13. *Instill the attitude that the body has a natural desire to heal.* Teach your children to trust in the innate natural wisdom of the body and its natural desire to be in healthy balance.

14. *Do everything you can to keep your children from smoking cigarettes.* And make sure they are not exposed to the tobacco smoke of others. Tobacco use is a major risk factor for cancer, heart disease, emphysema, and other serious long-term conditions, and those who start smoking the youngest have the most trouble quitting. And remember, passive exposure to Mom or Dad's cigarette smoke strongly contributes to allergies, ear infections, asthma, and other upper respiratory problems.

15. *Offer your unconditional love.* Give each child your full and undivided attention at some point every day.

16. *Be a good role model.* Be aware that the way you live your life is a lesson for your children. By taking good care of your own physical and mental health, you inspire your children to do the same.

CHAPTER 3

A Shot in the Arm (or the Leg):

Vaccinations

Shots! Now there's a word that can propel any child old enough to recognize it into a veritable tornado of activity designed to put off the inevitable. Bribery, bargaining, pleading, empty promises—we've heard it all. Fortunately, immunization methods are getting less painful, and children are incredibly forgiving. Not five minutes after having practically wrestled a kid to the ground to give him a shot, that same child will grab us around the knees and give us a big hug. And that's a good thing, because immunization against deadly disease is one of the first steps parents can take to protect their children's health.

We know that vaccination is a controversial topic in alternative medical circles, and it can be a source of tension between parents and the health professionals who care for their children. We think it's important for parents and physicians to be willing to engage in an honest dialogue on this issue. Our fervent hope is that these discussions will strengthen the parent-doctor relationship and ease parental fears about immunization. We hope parents will recognize that pediatricians are devoted to the health and safety of the children in their care and would not knowingly endanger them. For their part, physicians should recognize that questions from parents do not imply a lack of trust and that there are unanswered questions about vaccines that parents have a right—and a duty—to ask.

more on . . .

THE BENEFITS OF VACCINES

According to the Centers for Disease Control and Prevention (CDC), without vaccines we could expect each year:

- 13,000 to 20,000 cases of paralytic polio would occur, leaving thousands of children in braces or wheelchairs or dependent on ventilators.
- 600 kids would die from meningitis caused by *H. influenzae*, and many others would be left deaf or neurologically impaired.
- 7,500 or so would die from whooping cough, and close to 500 from measles.
- Pregnant women exposed to German measles (rubella) would suffer 2,100 stillbirths and deliver another 20,000 babies with heart defects, cognitive impairments, and/or deafness.

That said, we declare our bias up front. We are strongly in favor of immunizing your child. In fact, Dr. D is so convinced that immunization is vital to the health and safety of a child that in those rare cases when he cannot convince parents to immunize their children, he will drop the family from his practice. He feels that he cannot in good conscience allow children in his care to remain at risk for so many dangerous diseases.

A major advantage of integrative medicine is the ability to choose the safest, most effective treatments and protective practices from all the possibilities offered by conventional and alternative medicine. In this case we're going with conventional medical practice because we have seen the alternatives, and they are frightening to us as doctors and as fathers. When he was a young doctor training in the emergency room, Dr. Russ used to see many cases of bacterial meningitis, a bacterial infection of the fluid that surrounds the brain and spinal cord that laid previously healthy children so low so fast that they suffered terrible consequences if antibiotics were not administered immediately. Thanks to the *Haemophilus influenzae* (Hib) and *Pneumococcus* (Prevnar) vaccines, it's now uncommon for an emergency-department doctor to see this disease.

Similarly, Dr. D recalls the horror he experienced as a resident trying to ease the suffering of tiny patients with whooping cough (pertussis) as they struggled painfully for breath, choking and turning blue. The experience of knowing children who suffered and died of diseases that are now rare and preventable thanks to vaccines has thoroughly convinced us of the value of immunization.

Why Vaccinate?

The most compelling reason to immunize your child is that it works. That's why every state in the country requires certain shots before a child can enter the school system. Some diseases that were once common causes of childhood death or disability now appear rarely or never in this country. The widespread use of vaccines makes it possible for American parents to just take it for granted that their children will survive the infectious diseases of childhood. Parents in places where vaccines are not readily available don't have this luxury.

In addition to our concerns that each individual child be immunized, we also feel strongly that there is an important "common good" argument to be made for vaccinations. Immunization protects not just the person at the sharp end of the needle but also all the people with whom he or she comes in contact. Some people cannot be vaccinated themselves because of allergy, immune compromise, or fetal status, but when everyone else is vaccinated, the nonvaccinated benefit from the "herd immunity" created. We think that the socially responsible parent will also consider all the children who are too young or too ill to be immunized and act to protect them as well.

The campaign to wipe out German measles is a good example of the value of herd immunity. Its goal was the protection of pregnant women from exposure to rubella, which can cause birth defects. As a society we all get vaccinated against rubella because it drastically reduces exposure of pregnant women to the disease and insures that females carry some vaccine-induced antibodies to rubella in their system to protect future pregnancies.

National vaccine programs like this only work if there is a high level of participation. It is not enough to say that your kids don't have to be immunized because everyone else will be. Unfortunately, if enough people decide not to have their children immunized, a pool large enough to sustain an epidemic is created.

A temporary lapse in immunization practice from 1989 to 1991 led to pocket epidemics of measles in the United States that caused the preventable deaths of at least 120 people. Lapses in vaccination for whooping cough have led to its reappearance in some areas as well.

American children will need to continue vaccination programs even after some of these diseases become rare or extinct in the United States. Millions of people from other countries—many of them not fully immunized—come into the United States as either visitors or immigrants. Likewise, millions of Americans travel every year to countries where these diseases are more prevalent, and some of them return bearing pathogenic souvenirs.

Vaccine Facts

How Do Vaccines Work?

A vaccine, or immunization, is traditionally a weakened or killed form of a disease-causing virus or bacterium. Some of the newest vaccines are cloned from portions of the virus's genetic code that will provoke a similar immune response with fewer side effects. Some vaccines protect against a single disease, but others combine protection against two or three different diseases. When a vaccine is injected or swallowed or inhaled, it stimulates the formation of antibodies to the disease. These antibodies will target and attack the particular pathogen when they come across it later, preventing you from actually getting sick from the disease. In some cases a vaccine protects you completely. In other cases it protects you partially (you get only a mild form of the disease) or for only a certain length of time (which is why we have booster shots for diseases like tetanus).

The Diseases We Want to Prevent

We'd like to take a minute to acquaint you with the vaccines recommended by the Centers for Disease Control and the diseases they are designed to prevent:

DTaP (or TdaP for the booster shots needed by adults and children over ten). This combination vaccine provides protection from diphtheria, tetanus, and pertussis (whooping cough), three formerly common killers of children.

▶ *Diphtheria* is an aggressive bacterial infection that forms a choking membrane across the upper airway so a child cannot breathe. It also causes severe heart and nerve problems.

▶ *Tetanus* (lockjaw) is a muscular disorder caused by poisons generated when spores from a common soil bacterium enter the body through a wound. The spasms of tetanus are very painful and can become deadly if the muscles associated with breathing are affected.

▶ *Pertussis* usually just causes a mild cough in adults, but it can send a child into painful paroxysms of coughing that deprive the brain of oxygen and cause damage to the young infant's central nervous system.

MMR. This shot protects against measles, mumps, and rubella (German measles). Although these were once common childhood diseases—almost a rite of passage for your parents—they can be quite severe in adults, the immune compromised, or the very young.

▶ *Measles* can cause fatal encephalitis.

▶ *Mumps* can lead to sterility in males.

▶ *Rubella* can be devastating to developing fetuses, killing some in the womb and causing deafness, cognitive impairments, and heart problems in others.

Polio. This vaccine provides protection from a muscle-weakening virus, which, as late as the 1950s, was sentencing children and adults to wheelchairs and iron lungs. The oral vaccines containing weakened live virus protected the baby boomers, but in rare cases (six to seven cases a year in the United States and Canada) caused polio. Now children receive a safer, injectable vaccine made with inactivated poliovirus.

***Haemophilus influenzae* type b (Hib)**. This vaccine protects against the bacterium that most commonly causes meningitis in infants. During the 1980s, there were about seven thousand cases of Hib-related meningitis a year in children. Since introduction of the vaccine, cases of Hib have declined 98 percent.

Hepatitis B. This vaccine protects against an insidious, incurable, liver-damaging virus that is very easily transmissible. The earlier in life the disease is acquired, the more likely it is to be chronic and cause cirrhosis and liver cancer. Immunization as an infant protects against both infection during childhood and infection later in life from such risky behavior as unprotected sexual contact, piercing, injected drugs, etc.

Hepatitis A. This is a liver disease endemic in some parts of the country. While not usually a life-threatening disease, infection with hepatitis A can cause long and severe illness that is highly contagious.

Varicella. This vaccine protects against chicken pox, which is usually rather mild in children, but it is much more severe in adults or immunocompromised kids. However, when itchy kids scratch at their chicken pox, they create scores of portals for drug-resistant bacteria to enter and set up an infection that may be hard to cure. We once considered this vaccine optional, but with the increase in cases of drug-resistant bacteria such as methicillin-resistant *Staphylococcus aureus* (MRSA) in the community, we now strongly recommend it. Deaths from varicella-related infections have dropped two-thirds in this country since the introduction of this vaccine.

Pneumococcal conjugate. This vaccine is strongly recommended for all babies and for children at high risk for infections of the blood and brain caused by *Streptococcus pneumoniae*, such as kids with compromised immune systems, sickle-cell disease, or HIV infection. The vaccine also reduces the need for antibiotics by preventing the most resistant recurrent ear infections, as well as those most likely to lead to life-threatening meningitis. Use of this vaccine has led to an expected change in the type of bacteria that cause ear infections, but the newer inhabitants of the ear are less likely to cause serious invasive illness than *S. pneumoniae*.

Influenza. This vaccine is given annually for children under five because it drastically reduces the number of kids hospitalized with flu-related complications such as pneumonia. It is generally an injected vaccine, but there is also an inhaled version (FluMist) available. This intranasal version is free of thimerosal and provides slightly better immunity, but in Dr. D's experience, little children find it difficult to take and retain the vaccine without coughing.

Rotavirus. This infection causes potentially severe diarrhea in one in eight children under the age of two, especially those in day care. An earlier vaccine was pulled from use within twenty-four hours of reports it raised the risk for a serious intestinal obstruction. This problem has not occurred with the new oral vaccine, Rota Teq, which has been intensively studied.

Human Papillomavirus (HPV). This sexually transmitted virus has been linked to cervical cancer. Current recommendations are to immunize girls at age eleven to twelve, before they become sexually active. However, there are concerns that the protection against the virus may wear off before they actually do engage in sexual behavior, as well as concerns that the vaccine may not protect against all dangerous strains of the virus.

Meningitis. This can be especially dangerous when caused by a bacterium called *Neisseria meningitidis*. If *N. meningitidis* spreads throughout the body, it causes meningococcemia, a blood infection that can be rapidly fatal. People living in overcrowded situations—such as students in dormitories—are at increased risk of infection by *N. meningitidis*. That's why the meningococcal vaccine (Menactra) is currently required for preteens and adolescents aged eight through eighteen and recommended for those children aged two through ten at greater risk due to immune deficiencies, chronic disease, or attendance at summer camp.

Vaccine Safety

Many diligent parents have concerns about vaccines; some are legitimate, and some are based on misinformation. Your pediatrician or family practice doctor should be willing to listen and respond to these concerns thoughtfully and without judgment. You can also get excellent current information on vaccine safety from the National Immunization Program of the Centers for Disease Prevention and Control. (See Resources.)

more on . . .

ADULT VACCINES

Parents shouldn't neglect their own immunizations. Some childhood vaccines lose strength with time, requiring booster shots. New vaccines may offer protection not available when you were a child. Travel or medical conditions may require you to be immunized for illnesses that are not usually a problem for adults in this country. Ask your doctor to keep you up to date on your shots too.

Don't let anyone make you feel bad for asking questions about vaccines. In the past, such questions from doctors and parents have led to changes in some vaccine formulations and immunization schedules. For instance, the old vaccine for diphtheria, tetanus, and pertussis (DTP) has now been replaced by a new version (DTaP) that does not cause as many systemic side effects. (Although it may cause progressively worse local reactions with each shot, these are not long-lasting effects.) Similarly, when experience showed that the first children to get MMR vaccine appeared to lose their immunity around age twenty-five, a booster shot was added between ages four and six to maintain protection.

We cannot tell you that immunization is a 100 percent risk-free procedure—any medical intervention carries some degree of risk. Unlike early vaccines, though, today's vaccines have been more closely studied for safety and efficacy and carry fewer side effects. Currently vaccine safety is overseen by the Centers for Disease Prevention and Control (CDC), the National Institutes of Health (NIH), the American Committee for Immunization Practices (ACIP), the American Academy of Pediatrics (AAP), the National Vaccine Datalink Project, and the Food and Drug Administration (FDA).

Oddly, as vaccines improve, it sometimes seems like parental resistance to them has risen. Many parents still request exemption from the vaccinations required by their states for entry into school. All states provide medical exemption for children with allergies to the egg in flu vaccine or with a compromised immune system. A majority of states allow exemption for religious reasons, and some allow exemption for "philosophical" reasons as well.

The decision to avoid vaccination is gaining popularity largely because vaccines are so effective. It is clearly harder to make an informed decision about the risks versus the benefits of vaccines if parents have never seen the horrible effects of the diseases in question. If the disease is only an abstraction, the idea that there's a one in a million chance that your child could suffer a serious side effect from immunization tends to loom larger than the much higher risks of the disease itself. In addition, there's a public relations imbalance—the rare adverse effects of vaccines make the news, but the many deaths and impairments *prevented* by the vaccines are invisible. Here's one example. Despite headlines reporting that former Miss America Heather Whitestone's hearing impairment was a side effect of the whole-cell pertussis vaccine she'd been given as a child, her hearing loss was actually caused by a meningitis infection that today would have been prevented by the Hib vaccine.

more on . . .

VACCINE "COVER-UPS"

Once a vaccine is tested, approved by the FDA, and distributed, its effects are monitored closely, because side effects that may have escaped notice during clinical trials might become more obvious as larger groups of people experience them. This surveillance by several levels of government, pediatric associations, health maintenance organizations, and vaccine manufacturers is unceasing. A vaccine is monitored for as long as it is used. This system of multiple safeguards means that no single entity or organization has the power to impose the kind of cover-ups described by what we call "vaccine conspiracy theorists."

We frequently meet with parents who fear that vaccines might negatively impact their child's normal development. We acknowledge and address their concerns compassionately, but we still counsel that vaccination is the best course in all but the most unusual of circumstances. Is it possible that in rare instances a child may be predisposed to adverse, even long-term, responses to a vaccine? Yes. Is that reason enough not to vaccinate your children? Emphatically, no. Unfortunately, we cannot yet identify which children—if any—might be susceptible to these complications, but we already know that *all* children are at risk from the diseases these shots avert.

There's a wealth of good evidence that vaccination prevents illness and disability, saves lives, and does not contribute to developmental disorders like autism in healthy children. Parents and doctors all need to continue to push for even greater understanding of these complex issues, but ignoring the existing research does your children no benefit. As practitioners and fathers we eagerly await promised breakthroughs in genomics that may one day help identify the rare child who might be prone to vaccine complications. In the meantime, please vaccinate your children. It's the right thing to do.

Five Myths (and Two True Statements) about Vaccines

Let's look at the major concerns about vaccination one by one, evaluating the claims in the light of current research and our own medical experience. We don't have room to discuss any of these concerns in depth, so we will refer you to resources at the back of this book. But briefly, here are some of the common reasons given to withhold vaccination:

1. *The adverse effects of vaccines are worse than the disease themselves*. False.

According to the data collected by the Vaccine Adverse Effects Reporting System (VAERS) of the FDA, only *one death* was even possibly associated with the millions of shots given between 1990 and 1992. Even one death from vaccines is tragic, but many, many more children would have died of these diseases or their complications without immunization.

We have seen tens of thousands of children so far in our careers and have never seen a child with a permanent seizure or neurological side effects directly related to vaccination. Side effects are mild to nonexistent for the vast majority of children—nothing more than soreness at the site of the injection, rash, low-grade fever, and irritability. Rarely, seizures from high fever have been associated with measles vaccination, but these benign febrile seizures had no lasting effects. A serious muscular weakness called Guillain-Barré syndrome has been associated with the flu shot, but the risks of the disease are still substantially higher than the far rarer risks of the side effects.

2. *Too many vaccines too early in life damage the immune system*. False.

The first few months of life are when children are most at risk for these diseases because of their lack of natural immunity and inability to mount a strong immune response. For instance, pertussis may just cause a persistent cough in an adult, but it can cause brain damage if experienced before the age of six months. Giving the vaccine at a later age when the greatest risk for the disease has passed makes no sense.

The young immune system learns and becomes stronger by exposure to the milder forms of pathogens used in vaccines. Shots given in the first few months of life generally provide protection longer. Varicella vaccine, for example, does not "take" as well in children over twelve as it does in younger kids.

3. *We don't need all these vaccines anymore because the diseases are nearly eradicated in this country*. False.

Borders that look solid on the map are woefully inadequate to contain disease. Many of the diseases we consider nearly extinct are still alive and well in the developing world where lack of funds and lack of political will cripple attempts at general immunization. These diseases lurk at our doorstep, ready to be tracked in by the next traveler. We are also seeing some diseases reemerging as adult immunity to them wanes, so booster shots are important for both children and their parents.

4. *Measles/mumps/rubella (MMR) vaccine causes autism and inflammatory bowel disease*. False.

In 1998 a researcher in Great Britain reported a link between MMR inoculation and these two disorders, and vaccine antagonists there immediately began demanding the withdrawal of the vaccine. The study was later discredited and withdrawn when investigation proved that research data had been falsified or slanted and that money and participants for the study had been supplied by a law firm suing vaccine manufacturers. Larger studies by others have consistently found *no difference* in the rate of autism before and after the introduction of the MMR vaccine. However, publicity about the study caused a drop in MMR vaccine participation that has led to epidemics of measles in Great Britain and Israel.

5. *Some vaccines contain toxic mercury*. True, with caveats.

In 1999 it was discovered that infants could possibly accumulate more than the level of mercury considered safe by the FDA if all the vaccines they were given in their first year contained the mercury-based preservative thimerosal. Although thimerosal has been used for decades to prevent bacterial contamination of vaccines with no apparent ill effects, the compound was removed from most vaccines given to children as a safety measure. We do suggest that parents ask for vaccines free of thimerosal for their children, as they are now readily available. Studies consistently find no support for the claim that thimerosal causes autism, and, in fact, autism rates continued to go up even after thimerosal was removed.

6. *Combination vaccines are more dangerous than single vaccines*. False.

The primary question about the "super-combination" vaccines that administer four or more vaccines at once was not one of safety so much as effectiveness. However, studies have found that combination vaccines are actually safer, more effective, and have fewer side effects than single vaccines, while reducing the number of times a child has to be poked with a needle and the cost to the parent.

7. *Vaccines do not completely protect you from disease*. True.

No vaccine offers 100 percent protection, because individual responses to vaccines vary. Most vaccines offer about 90 percent efficacy at outset. With time, some individuals lose some of this immunity. For instance, 5 percent of children vaccinated for chicken pox will develop a mild case of the disease if exposed to the virus later. However, most vaccines protect you during the time period when you are most at risk, and almost all vaccines lessen the severity of the disease should you happen to contract it despite immunization.

Our Vaccine Recommendations

We generally suggest that parents follow the recommendations of the CDC or the American Academy of Pediatrics regarding immunizations. The AAP takes a very activist approach to vaccines and vaccine safety, and we trust them to consider the safety of our children as a group and as individuals.

All vaccine guidelines give a range of time when a vaccine can be given, and we think they should be adhered to as much as possible. Sometimes parents request that we split the MMR vaccine into its separate components, but we now find this to be a bad practice. It makes achieving optimal immunity more difficult, as well as increasing the number of shots and office visits required (and decreasing full compliance).

The following chart gives a simplified version of the current AAP recommendations as of the date of publication of this book:

YEAR ONE	YEAR TWO	YEAR FOUR AND AFTER
DTaP (diphtheria/tetanus/pertussis) at 2 months, 4 months, and 6 months	**DTaP** at 15 to 18 months	**DTaP** at 4 to 6 years, **TdaP** at 11 to 12 years, and **tetanus** boosters every 10 years thereafter
Polio at 2 months, 4 months, and 6 to 18 months		**Polio** at 4 to 6 years
MMR (measles/mumps/rubella) at 12 to 15 months		**MMR** at 4 to 6 years
Hepatitis B at birth and 2 more doses within first year		
Varicella (chicken pox) at 12 to 15 months	**Varicella** at 18 months	
Hib (*H. influenzae*) at 2 and 4 months	**Hib** at 12 to 15 months	
Pneumococcal at 2, 4, and 6 months	**Pneumococcal** at 12 to 15 months if child did not receive it as an infant	
Rotavirus at 2, 4, and 6 months	2 doses 6 months apart at 15 to 18 months	
Hepatitis A		
Meningococcal		once at age 11 to 12, one more at age 15 to 17
Influenza at 6 months	once annually	once annually
Human Papillomavirus (HPV), linked to cervical cancer		3 doses in 6 months starting any time age 11 to 23

When Not to Give a Shot

We rarely hold off giving a vaccine just because a child has a cold. We do hold off on giving the MMR, varicella, and nasal flu vaccines to a child with the sniffles, because viral infections may reduce the immune response to a live, attenuated-virus vaccine. We do not give a scheduled shot if a child has a fever over 101 degrees; we may delay a shot in children with milder fevers if the parent seems especially worried about it. We don't give flu shots to kids with egg allergy. They can receive an MMR but should remain in the office for observation for a short period of time afterward. Children taking immunosuppressive drugs have modified immunization schedules.

Easing the Aftereffects

Some vaccines will cause slight side effects, such as swelling, itching, or redness at the site of the injection, a mild fever, or irritability. *Call the doctor* if your child displays a more serious response such as high fever, persistent screaming, or seizure. If unable to reach the doctor, consider a trip to the emergency department.

There are a few ways to reduce the mild side effects of inoculations.

- Ask the doctor to massage the site of the injection for thirty seconds before giving the injection. Children tend to find this soothing.
- Calm your child by rocking, stroking, speaking in a soothing voice, or giving a pacifier or a favorite toy. Such distractions reduce infant distress with the injections.
- Consider a brief session of hypnotherapy beforehand to make the experience more pleasant.
- Lower your own levels of anxiety so your child does not pick up on your tension and become tense too. Treat vaccination matter-of-factly and your kids will too.

- Use children's acetaminophen after an injection to reduce soreness at the injection site.
- Apply a cold compress. Toss a clean wet washcloth in the freezer. An hour later you'll have an easy-to-use cold compress to reduce any inflammation or pain at the injection site.
- Try a topical anesthetic at the injection site.

CHAPTER 4

Drugs and Bugs:

The Proper Use of Antibiotics

The development of antibiotic drugs may be the single greatest medical achievement of the twentieth century. After penicillin became available during World War II, the number of deaths from bacterial infections dropped so sharply that few people today realize how dangerous many diseases—even common ones like strep throat and pneumonia—once were. Unfortunately, these "miracle drugs" were so effective as weapons against disease-causing bacteria that they were also seen as a cure-all for almost any condition. By now we have so abused antibiotic drugs that the miracle has turned into something of a mixed blessing.

Over the past few decades it has become more and more obvious that by misusing and overusing antibiotics we have weakened their effectiveness, creating new strains of "superbugs" that are highly resistant to many drugs. In our practices we now see hard-to-treat diseases caused by these highly aggressive bacteria, diseases we have never seen before. We find this development so worrisome—and the need to educate parents so great—that we are devoting an entire chapter to antibiotics.

Antibiotic ABCs

The term *antibiotic* refers to a drug that kills or inhibits bacteria. Antibiotics do not kill viruses, so—contrary to popular belief—they are useless against viral diseases like colds, influenza, and most other viral upper respiratory infections.

The first of the widely available antibiotics were sulfonamide and penicillin. There are now more than a hundred antibiotics available, including tetracyclines, cephalosporins, quinolones, and macrolides. Those that work only against certain categories of germs are called *narrow-spectrum antibiotics.* Those that have actions against a wider variety of microbes are called *broad-spectrum antibiotics.*

The Dark Side of Antibiotic Drugs

There has always been a dark side to antibiotics. Alexander Fleming, the man who discovered penicillin, noted that greater exposure to the drug caused the targeted bacteria to mutate—and become harder to kill. In the inevitable process of natural selection, the most susceptible strains of targeted bacteria are destroyed, leaving the hardier ones to survive and evolve new defenses against the drug's next attack. The mutated bacteria can pass their resistance on to their "children" and to unrelated bacteria within hours of exposure to a strong antibiotic. These resistant bacteria cause more severe, less treatable infections that require higher doses of drugs, combinations of drugs, or new drugs altogether, to which—inevitably—the bacteria also adapt.

When antibiotics are used properly, the progression of antibiotic attack and bacterial adaptation goes more slowly, so it takes time to build up complete bacterial resistance to a drug. But we have sped up the course of events by our overuse of the drugs. It took five years for the first strains of bacteria resistant to penicillin to show up. Resistance to the newest antibiotic drugs may already be seen in a drug's preapproval trials.

In 1954 manufacturers produced two million pounds of antibiotic drugs; 50 years later they produce (and we use) more than 25 times that amount. Americans get about three times more antibiotic prescriptions per person than people in more antibiotic-wary European countries like the Netherlands. And lots of those prescriptions are useless. The Centers for Disease Control and Prevention estimates that almost half of all outpatient prescriptions for antibiotics are given for viral diseases not affected by antibiotics.

more on . . .
BACTERIAL RESISTANCE

According to Dr. Stuart Levy of Tufts University, founder of the Alliance for the Prudent Use of Antibiotics, five underlying principles of bacterial resistance cause concern:

1. Antibiotic resistance is inevitable, given enough time and enough drugs used.
2. Bacteria evolve to become progressively more resistant to a drug.
3. Bacteria that are resistant to one drug are likely to become resistant to others.
4. Bacteria lose this resistance slowly, if at all.
5. Resistant bacteria are easily transmitted from one person to another.

Our overexposure to antibiotics—from prescription medicines, antibacterial products (such as soaps), and veterinary drugs in our food—is causing a frightening increase in the number of strains of bacteria resistant to all but one or two antibiotic drugs. Until recently, medical science dealt with the increased resistance of bacteria and reduced effectiveness of drugs by building bigger and stronger antibiotics (a microbial version of the arms race). Of course, as these second- and third-generation drugs were used more frequently, bacteria become wise to them as well. Basically, modern pharmaceutical technology has created a "cure" for disease that insures the survival of a more evolved disease-causing organism.

It's ironic that improper use of the greatest medical discovery of the twentieth century has put the children and adults of the twenty-first century at risk. We have inadvertently created so many strains of bacteria that are invulnerable to drugs that researchers are scrambling to find new classes of antibiotics. Similar resistance is developing to antifungal and antiviral drugs.

The strains of bacteria that develop resistance vary geographically, depending on the particular prescribing and practice habits of doctors and hospitals in the area. What is resistant in one geographic area may be easily treated in another, although there is evidence that some of the resistant strains are spreading to far-flung corners of the globe. Most of the nastier strains of resistant bacteria are more commonly found in institutions such as hospitals and nursing homes, where there are large numbers of people with lowered immunity getting multiple drugs. However, some of these new bacteria are now showing up in healthy people, causing serious bacterial infections. It is no longer rare to hear of healthy young adults succumbing to a bacterial infection.

What Are We Doing Wrong?

Resistant strains of bacteria are arising more rapidly for at least six reasons:

- *Antibiotics are overprescribed.* Millions of prescriptions for antibiotics are issued for colds, influenza, and other viral conditions for which they are worthless. Other times prescriptions aren't necessary in the short term (such as early in the course of ear infections, sinusitis, or bronchitis) or turn out not to be effective in the long term (such as use of antibiotics to prevent recurrent urinary tract infections).

- *Antibiotics are used improperly by patients.* We all know people who stop taking a prescription as soon as they start to feel better, despite the doctor's orders to continue for a week to ten days. Not taking the complete dose of an antimicrobial has the unfortunate effect of killing off those bacteria most susceptible to the drug and leaving the strongest to survive, thrive, and possibly mutate to a form that does not respond to the drug. You get the same result when you use "leftover" pills to inadequately self-medicate another condition later.

- *Antibiotics are used improperly by health professionals.* Health professionals who give in to parents begging for antibiotics or who routinely begin with broad-spectrum antibiotics set the stage for more kinds of bacteria to develop resistance. It's better to start with the narrowest and least expensive forms of antibiotics and switch over to more complex broader-spectrum drugs only if there is no clinical improvement over the first 48–72 hours.

- *Antibacterial products are overused.* Antibacterial soaps or other products don't actually reduce the risk for infectious disease in healthy families, but regular exposure to these unnecessary antibiotics does increase bacterial resistance.

▶ *More children attend day care.* Children who play together eventually share all the coexisting bacteria they each carry. This exposure has the benefit of helping train the developing immune system. It is also the reason why children in day care and nursery programs acquire new infections all the time and why some parents of school-age children wryly refer to them as "living incubators." If children within those small groups develop resistant bacteria, they are shared by every member of the group, and eventually with everyone with whom they come in contact.

▶ *More people are exposed to antibiotics secondhand through meat and dairy products.* Many of the antibiotics fed to food animals in low doses to speed growth or in higher doses to treat infections are passed on to us in food. Giving growth-promoting antibiotics at sub-therapeutic levels—that is, at dosages insufficient to wipe the bacteria out—is a virtual recipe for creating resistant bacteria.

more on . . .

MRSA

Methicillin-resistant *Staphylococcus aureus* (MRSA) is one of the superbugs now found not just in hospitals and institutions but also in living rooms, locker rooms, and classrooms. It is usually treatable, but is most dangerous in the very young, the very old, and the very sick—and occasionally is lethal even in the healthy. MRSA is transmitted through skin-to-skin contact, so good hygiene is important. Among the ways the Centers for Disease Control suggest you reduce your risk for MRSA:

- ▶ Wash hands frequently with regular soap.
- ▶ Avoid overuse or misuse of antibiotics.
- ▶ Cover open wounds with a dry bandage.
- ▶ Don't share razors, towels, or other personal items.
- ▶ Shower well after sports, especially those that include contact with people or equipment.

Getting Back on the Right Track

As the problems that can be associated with these drugs have become more obvious, major campaigns for reducing antibiotic resistance have been launched by the National Academy of the Sciences, the CDC, the American Academy of Pediatrics, and the American Medical Association. These national campaigns to reduce antibiotic use are focusing not just on physicians but on the public as well. Physicians like us who take a measured approach to antibiotics already spend a lot of time educating parents about the reasons for this practice, but parents have to do their part too. For instance:

- *Don't be overly concerned if we don't recommend antibiotics immediately for a low-grade infection.* A wait-and-see approach often gives the body time to heal itself.
- *Don't demand the broadest-spectrum antibiotics available for the simplest of infections.* Some parents want the stronger drugs because, they say, "My child doesn't respond to amoxicillin." The important thing to remember is that children are not resistant to antibiotics—bacteria are! Lack of response to antibiotics is not a function of the child's immune system but rather a function of the bacterial strain. Or it may be that the cause is a virus against which antibiotics have no efficacy.
- *Don't demand antibiotics for a viral infection.* Antibiotics don't kill viruses. Unfortunately, since colds and the flu generally run their course and clear up on their own, people who take antibiotics for them attribute their recovery to the drug and insist on a prescription every time they start to sniffle.

Doctors often react to this actual or perceived parental pressure by prescribing antibiotics even when they know there will be no medical benefit, especially if they have free samples from the pharmaceutical companies to eliminate cost from the equation. If this kind of thinking doesn't change, we won't have effective antibiotics when we really need them.

Our Antibiotic Practices

As integrative practitioners, we are committed to supporting natural efforts to heal. We know that invading organisms sometimes slip through our natural defenses and set off a bacterial infection. When this happens, the immune system usually just goes to work and clears up the problem with no need for drugs. But sometimes—because the bacteria are particularly strong or reproducing especially fast, or because the immune system is not functioning at peak efficiency—our natural defenses are overwhelmed. This is when we turn to antibiotics, because these drugs can reduce the numbers of the bacteria enough for the immune system to be able to take over and heal the infection. We look at antibiotics not necessarily as a cure on their own but as an aid to the immune response. This is a very different philosophical perspective from that of conventional doctors.

A cautious approach to antibiotics will not leave your child at the mercy of every bacterium that crosses his path. Children are remarkably resilient creatures and usually bounce back quickly from the transient stress of an infection. Whenever possible, and where clinically appropriate, we try to wait and give our patients' little bodies a chance to muster their own defenses before charging in with the big antibiotic guns.

Although antibiotics can be very useful, they are not completely benign drugs. The main side effect of antibiotics in children is diarrhea and gastrointestinal upset, as the drug alters the natural balance of bacterial flora in the bowel. These drugs also carry the potential for allergic reactions, both mild and severe. Parents also report to us that some kids taking antibiotics act "very weird," with greater irritability, more crying, and more misbehavior.

That inherent American desire for a quick fix makes our more cautious way of addressing childhood infections a tough sell at first, but our good results speak for themselves. We take the time to explain the reasons for not immediately prescribing antibiotics and decide—together with the parents—which tactic to follow. We may decide on a period of watchful waiting if the parents are willing to monitor their child's progress, call in if the child's symptoms worsen, and schedule a follow-up visit three to seven days later to check that the infection has resolved. We may respond more conservatively (with a prescription for an antibiotic) when careful follow-up is not likely to occur.

more on . . .
BACTERIAL ECOLOGY

There are more than 100 trillion bacteria in your body, with more than two pounds of them in your colon alone. Gut bacteria digest your food, make vitamins K and B12, protect you from more dangerous bacteria, send signals that affect body function, turn specific genes on or off, and influence the immune system in the gut and in the body as a whole. Interfering with the natural bacterial ecology of the body—whether through antibiotic use, diet, or stress—can create a minor yeast infection, a major overgrowth of a germ like *C. difficile*, or changes in bowel habits, or even alter the proper function of the immune system in a way that leads to inflammation.

Sometimes parents are determined to get an antibiotic for their child because they have come to think of the word *antibiotic* as a synonym for "strong, effective medicine." In those cases we might offer them a prescription but ask that they wait a day or two to see if the condition worsens before filling it. With a prescription reassuringly in hand, most parents are more willing to wait to see if the problem clears up on its own. A good relationship between parents and physician is essential here, as the physician must be able to trust the parents' oversight of the situation and the parent must be able to trust that the physician will respond quickly if needed.

In general, we tend to prescribe older antibiotic drugs like amoxicillin because they are more narrowly targeted, rather than the hotly marketed new drugs, which we save for more serious infections. Narrow-spectrum drugs engender resistance in fewer types of bacteria.

TIP: Parents who are monitoring their children during a "wait-and-see" period should call the child's physician and start prescribed antibiotic treatment at these signs: worsening pain, fussiness or other atypical behavior, decreased intake of solids and especially liquids, reduced urine output, persistent vomiting, or difficulties with breathing.

Taking Advantage of Probiotics

When we do prescribe systemic or oral antibiotics we often also prescribe a complementary course of what are called *probiotics* (or "good bacteria") to help maintain a healthy balance of bacteria in the large intestine. The bowel normally contains hundreds of strains of bacteria, many of them necessary to the proper function of the body. Some of these bacteria can cause disease themselves, but other bacteria normally keep them in check. Unfortunately, antibiotics cannot tell a good bug from a bad one in the dark and may upset the healthy balance of the bacterial flora in a way that causes diarrhea in 20 to 40 percent of all children prescribed antibiotics, and vaginal yeast infections in some girls.

Probiotics are microorganisms that can exert health benefits above and beyond basic nutrition. Probiotic foods or supplements are used to replace one or more of the beneficial intestinal bacteria that might normally be killed by an antibiotic. Probiotic foods include yogurt with active cultures, kefir, naturally fermented pickles, kim chee, and dairy products fortified with various strains of bacteria, including *Lactobacillus* or *Bifidobacterium*. A frequent probiotic prescription is either one cup of yogurt with active cultures a day or a probiotic supplement taken as directed throughout the course of antibiotics and for a week thereafter.

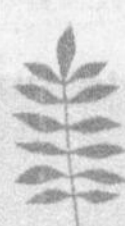

TIP: Prebiotics are non-absorbable sugars such as fructo-oligosaccharides that healthy gut bacteria prefer as food. Products that contain both probiotic microbes and the prebiotic ingredients that help them flourish are called symbiotics.

Powdered and chewable probiotic supplements are also available for kids. Some have significant strain-specific research supporting their use, but many others have been found unworthy of the claims made for them. You can increase your odds of getting an effective product that will still be viable when it gets to the large intestine by looking for an enteric-coated supplement that contains at least 10 billion colony-forming units (CFU) of the named microbe or symbiotic. Supplements containing lactobacilli and bifidobacteria have been proven in recent studies to greatly reduce both the incidence and the duration of diarrhea caused by antibiotics and may even help prevent certain illnesses such as eczema, recurrent C. *difficile* infection, and viral diarrheal illness.

What Parents Can Do

We believe the concerted efforts at patient and physician education now taking place in this country will help preserve the usefulness of antibiotics. Here are nine ways to do your part:

1. *Don't pressure your doctor for antibiotic drugs*. Don't request antibiotics for viral infections like colds and flu or suspected viral infections. Give mild conditions a few days to heal on their own. Even if antibiotics have appeared to be helpful in the past, keep in mind that your child might have healed just as quickly without them.

2. *If your child's doctor prescribes antibiotics, make sure you understand the rationale behind the prescription*. Studies have found that pediatricians often think a parent wants a child to get an antibiotic when in fact the parent just wants the child to feel better.

3. *Indicate your openness to a wait-and-see policy when appropriate*.

4. *Use antibiotics as prescribed*. Don't stop taking them before you should, and don't use leftover antibiotics or someone else's prescription.

5. *Keep track of your family's usage of antibiotics*. That way you know what drugs have been used and to what effect. Make sure anyone caring for your child knows about any allergies to antibiotics your child may have.

6. *Buy organic meats and dairy products that are free of antibiotics if finances allow*. Lobby for government restriction of antibiotic use in food animals.

7. *Train your children to wash their hands frequently*. Make sure that their preschools and schools allow/encourage hand washing as well. It's an easy way to reduce diarrhea, respiratory infections, and urinary tract infections. If your child's school is suffering an outbreak of infectious disease, check the restrooms to make sure they are adequately stocked with soap and paper towels.

more on . . .
HAND WASHING

Hygiene experts say we need soap, water, and at least twenty seconds to get hands clean. How long is twenty seconds? Two choruses of either "Happy Birthday" or "Wheels on the Bus." Maybe you can get your kids to hum as they rub their soapy palms together briskly, interlace fingers, rub them quickly up and down, and scrub under their nails.

8. *Avoid the use of antibacterial soaps, toys, blankets, etc.* According to the CDC, plain soap and water are just as effective as the heavily advertised antibacterial soaps and have the additional advantage of not encouraging the growth of resistant bacteria.

9. *Make sure your children get the recommended vaccinations*. It's a lot better to prevent infections than to have to treat them with antibiotics.

CHAPTER 5

The Joy of Eating:

Healthy Eating Patterns for Life

Once upon a time the dining room table was the heart of the home, a place where friends and family gathered together to enjoy a home-cooked meal, share stories, and express gratitude for the gifts of life. Dinner was a time of connection and relaxation, not a forced refueling stop in a busy day, a time to watch the news, or a place to play out various food obsessions. Other cultures still stress the social aspect of dining, but the ability to savor food and family sometimes seems lost—or maybe just mislaid—in our own country.

Studies have consistently shown that kids who regularly eat meals with their families have a healthier diet, enjoy closer family relationships, do better in school, show less stress, suffer less depression, get into less trouble with the law, and are less likely to use tobacco, drugs, or alcohol. Yet according to a 2003 Gallup Poll, only 28 percent of families with children under eighteen make it a point to eat together every night. And the two-thirds of American families who keep the TV on during dinner at least some of the time may be sharing the same space, but they're probably not sharing the events of their days with one another over the blare of the TV.

Despite our best intentions, our own experiences tend to back up these statistics. Mealtimes at our homes are sometimes rushed occasions squeezed in between school, work, Scouts, sports, dance class, and other activities. The plates at our tables are sometimes filled with takeout food or a processed meal tossed in the microwave. We have seen our own pleasant family meals deteriorate into arguments over how much and what types of food our kids are willing to eat. We know it's difficult to serve healthy food that our kids will eat with pleasure when every day it seems there is a new "food villain" to worry about. We know. We know. We've got eight kids among us, and we've been there.

We want to help you bring the pleasure back to eating. We are going to explain the basics of a healthy diet without creating categories of irredeemably "bad" foods or making every "good" food sound like a medical prescription. We are also going to give you the information that will allow you to counter the unhealthy commercial and cultural messages about food that assault your children day in and day out.

Let's start by looking at the reality of how today's kids eat. Of children between the ages of one and nine, 99 percent do not meet the federal guidelines for a healthy diet. Most children eat only one serving of vegetables a day, often french fries. Very few of them get anywhere near the amount of calcium they need to build strong bones and teeth for life. They eat increasing amounts of snacks high in sugar, salt, and fat, and drink more and more sugary beverages. (These highly processed foods are not only full of empty calories, but they may also interfere with the absorption of real nutrients.) And they take in too many calories for their activity levels.

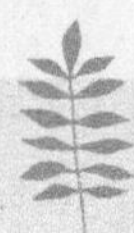

TIP: The government recommends your child get 6 to 11 servings of grains, 3 to 5 servings of vegetables, 2 to 4 servings of fruit, and 2 to 3 servings of dairy products a day.

Is it any wonder that the number of children who are overweight has doubled in the past thirty years? Like their parents, our children are eating too much and exercising too little, causing an epidemic of obesity in America. We will discuss obesity in children more in chapter 6, but we want to make sure that you understand that your growing child's diet can have long-term effects—good or ill—on your child's health as an adult. The seeds of such serious medical problems as adult obesity, cardiovascular disease, diabetes, osteoporosis, stroke, and probably some cancers are sown during childhood. That's why it is essential for you to encourage good nutritional habits now that will serve your child for a lifetime.

On the flip side of this obesity epidemic is the fact that one in six children live in households that struggle to meet their basic food needs. Nearly a third of households headed by a single woman are considered to be "food insecure." This malnourishment has long-term implications as well, because deficiencies in important nutrients can affect both health and educational attainments. It has also been implicated as a potential contributing factor in criminal behavior. It is essential that we all work to insure that the breakfasts and lunches provided for free at public schools be as nutritious as possible, especially since they may be the only meals that many children eat all day.

There is no way that we can cover nutrition from birth to age twelve in one chapter and be anywhere near as thorough as we'd like to be. If you are interested in a fuller discussion of nutrition, check out our resources section. In the meantime, here's our overview.

Prenatal Nutrition

By now, everyone knows the importance of good prenatal nutrition. It's clear that pregnant women who don't eat well are more likely to give birth to children with low birth weight, physical defects, and potential intellectual and behavioral deficits. But what has only recently been discovered is how much a pregnant woman's diet may affect her child's health into *adulthood*. Recent research suggests that the stage may be set in the womb for cardiovascular disease, diabetes, high cholesterol, and other serious conditions of adulthood.

The developing fetus is especially vulnerable during the first trimester of pregnancy. In those first three months—during part of which the woman does not even realize she is pregnant—the spinal cord and central nervous system take form. Because it is particularly important to have an adequate supply of the B vitamin folic acid during this period to prevent neural tube birth defects such as spina bifida, we recommend that all women of childbearing age get at least 800 mcg (micrograms) of folic acid every day through fortified foods or a multivitamin.

Later in the pregnancy, other nutrients become important. For instance, a pregnant woman must get enough calcium (1,200 to 1,500 mg) and iron (30 mg) a day for two, so that her own stocks of these nutrients won't become depleted as her fetus builds bones, teeth, and the iron stores that will help tide the baby over for the first four to six months of life (breast milk is low in iron). She should also make sure to get a total intake of 1,000 IU a day of vitamin D (in the form of cholecalciferol), especially if she is dark skinned or pregnant during the winter months when she is less likely to get enough vitamin D from sunlight. Low fetal levels of vitamin D are associated with preeclampsia during childbirth as well as bone and growth problems in the babies.

Throughout your pregnancy it's important to eat a varied diet with enough calories—about 300 more calories a day than usual. You want to gain 25 to 35 pounds with your pregnancy, to increase the chances that your baby will be born at a healthy weight. Focus on high-quality foods like whole grains, produce of all types, lean meats, beans, and low-fat dairy foods.

Do include more foods high in omega-3 fatty acids, such as walnuts and ground flaxseed. The latest research is showing the possibility of a connection between omega-3 fatty acids taken in by mothers and proper brain and visual development in their infants. We don't recommend that pregnant women eat fish itself because of the environmental toxins it may contain, but we do recommend that pregnant and nursing women take 2 g a day of a purified (mercury-free) fish oil.

Ask your doctor if any of the herbs, dietary supplements, or medications you're currently taking can affect your unborn child. We don't recommend adding any new supplements except prenatal vitamins, fish oil, and any supplemental vitamin D needed to reach a 1,000 IU a day level. A probiotic supplement taken by a pregnant woman in the latter half of the third trimester and given to a newborn for the first few months of life may help prevent the development of allergic disorders such as eczema.

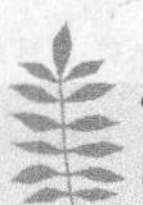

TIP: If you do crave fish while pregnant, eat only wild (not farmed) salmon or no more than 6 ounces a week of skipjack (not albacore) tuna.

We encourage pregnant women to drink purified drinking water, wash their produce, avoid food microwaved in plastic containers, and eat organic food when available and affordable to lessen their exposure to environmental pollutants. We are especially concerned about the potential for subtle nervous system and hormonal disturbances in children born to mothers exposed to the hormonally active agents found in pesticides, polychlorinated biphenyls (PCBs), and dioxins. (See chapter 8.)

SUMMARY OF PRENATAL NUTRITION

- Take prenatal vitamins once you decide to get pregnant.
- Make sure you get enough calcium, vitamin D, and iron.
- Get enough good calories.
- Take a daily fish oil supplement for omega-3 fatty acids. Avoid fish.
- Do not use alcohol or tobacco.

Feeding Your Child to Age Two

Breast-Feeding

We believe strongly that children should be breast-fed until they are at least one year of age. We understand that this isn't possible for all women, such as those taking certain medications, but the research is clear that breast-feeding is optimal. If you cannot or simply choose not to breast-feed your child, however, don't worry that it will ruin your relationship with your baby. Despite the dogmatic insistence of some organized advocates for breast-feeding, it is not the only way to form a close bond with a new child.

Breast-feeding offers real benefits to both mother and child. For baby, it:

- Provides maternal antibodies while the baby's own immune system is developing

- Reduces the incidence of diarrhea, upper respiratory infections, ear infections, and other bacterial and viral illnesses

- Lowers the chances of developing chronic digestive disorders and some childhood cancers and may lessen the incidence of allergies and asthma

- Protects against obesity and type-1 diabetes in childhood

- Protects against cardiovascular problems and type-2 diabetes in adulthood

- May increase intelligence

- Provides a stronger beneficial response to immunization

- Is more digestible than formula, is a more efficient source of energy, and provides hundreds of compounds such as growth factors, hormones, and essential fatty acids not found in infant formulas

For mother, breast-feeding:

- May reduce the risk of breast and ovarian cancer in premenopausal women

- Saves money and time on formula

- Speeds postpartum healing of the uterus

- Burns 500 extra calories a day so you can get back into your jeans faster

Even with all these advantages, only 68 percent of American women even try nursing, and only 19 percent nurse their babies for a full year—one of the lowest rates for breast-feeding in the world. Perhaps this is because we don't provide enough education and support for nursing mothers. New mothers are generally discharged from the hospital within 24 hours of giving birth, so few of them have a chance to learn how to breast-feed in a relaxed and comforting atmosphere. In addition, few employers provide private space for breast pumping, and most Americans still feel uncomfortable around any woman who, even discreetly, raises her blouse to feed her infant. Despite promotion of breast-feeding by the federal government and the American Academy of Pediatrics, Americans do not yet view nursing as a natural activity.

If you are having trouble nursing, ask your primary care physician for a referral to a lactation specialist. Four important factors lead to breast-feeding success:

1. *Good nutrition*. You'll need about 2,500 calories a day to make milk high enough in the fatty acids so important to your child's growth and development.

2. *Lots of liquids*. Drink at least eight glasses of water a day to keep your milk flowing.

3. *Plenty of rest*. A fatigued or anxious mother may produce less milk, and her baby may develop poor nursing patterns—such as a weak suck or spitting up—that lead to low weight gain. Make rest a priority. Remember the "in-flight oxygen mask" rule cited by every flight attendant in the world: Take care of yourself first, so you can care for your children.

4. *Support from family and friends*. Ignore the dusty tabletops, cut back on work or volunteer responsibilities if you can, and ask for help from friends and family. You're not being selfish—you're being a good mother.

At three to four months of age, breast-fed infants should be started on infant vitamin/mineral supplement drops to provide additional amounts of iron and vitamin D. This is especially important for dark-skinned infants, who do not absorb vitamin D as well from the sun.

TIP: What you eat can affect your baby's digestion and mood. If you think your diet may be causing colic or fussiness, try eliminating a suspect food for a few days to see if it makes a difference. If you cut dairy, add a calcium supplement to make sure you get enough of this mineral essential to a nursing mother.

Formula

If you will not be breast-feeding your child, you will need to choose an infant formula. Regular cow's milk is not an option, as it can cause gastrointestinal bleeding and iron deficiency in children under a year of age.

There are basically three categories of formula: milk (casein) based, soy based, and "predigested" formulas for children with allergies or significant gastroesophageal reflux (vomiting and spitting up). All have been developed to match human breast milk as closely as possible. We generally recommend milk-based formulas such as Similac or Enfamil, which are well tolerated by most babies. Be sure to get formula with added DHA (docosahexaenoic acid) or other forms of omega-3 fatty acids, which appear to help with brain development. If you can find and afford organic infant formula, that would be our first choice.

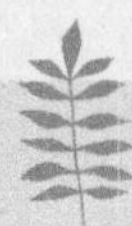

TIP: Avoid liquid formula sold in cans lined with a hormone-disrupting chemical called bisphenol A (BPA), and opt for formula in plastic or BPA-free containers instead.

Solid Foods

You may begin to introduce solid foods to formula-fed infants at about four months of age. You'll want to wait longer with breast-fed babies—until about six or seven months—as they may suck less strongly and take in less breast milk once they start eating solids. Our advice is to start with a simple bland food like iron-fortified rice cereal, and slowly add other foods, one at a time, so you can more easily identify the cause of any food allergy that might show up in the form of skin disorders, recurrent respiratory tract infections, or gastrointestinal problems.

We recommend that you move to vegetables after rice cereal, starting with red/orange ones like squash and sweet potatoes, then moving to green ones like peas and string beans. Fruits would come next. We hold off on introducing berries, peanuts, egg whites (yolks are okay after nine months), and other frequently allergenic foods until a child is at least a year old. Yogurt, cottage cheese, and pureed meats can be added after seven months.

You can buy pureed foods or make them yourself with a portable food grinder or food mill. Dr. D's wife used to prepare several meals' worth at once by pureeing the foods into ice cube trays and defrosting as needed. Do not feed babies younger than seven months homemade pureed carrots, beets, turnips, spinach, or collard greens because in some parts of the country (generally agricultural areas) these vegetables are too high in nitrates for a very young child. Commercial manufacturers screen for nitrates, so their products are safe at any age. If you buy commercial baby foods, make sure they contain low levels of added salt, sugar, and other fillers, and look for the organic products offered by several manufacturers. Avoid purees of highly allergic fruits like strawberries and kiwi in the first year.

As far as first beverages go, when your child is old enough for regular soy or cow's milk (over twelve months), give her pasteurized, organic full-fat milks until fifteen months, when you can switch to skim or nonfat milk. In contrast to adults, babies need plenty of fat in their first two years, as fat fuels the creation of brain tissue. We hope you won't introduce fruit juice during a child's first year and are cautious with the amount of fruit juice you allow your child thereafter. Excessive intake of fruit juice can cause gastrointestinal problems and tooth decay or be a contributing factor in failure to gain weight in the second year of life.

SUMMARY TO AGE TWO

- ▶ Breast-feed your child for a full year if at all possible.
- ▶ If you use formula, try a milk-based (casein) one first.
- ▶ Do not feed liquid cow's milk to children under a year of age.
- ▶ At three or four months, start breast-fed babies on an infant supplement that provides at least vitamin D and iron.
- ▶ Introduce solid foods to formula-fed infants at about four months of age, to breast-fed babies at six to seven months of age.
- ▶ Hold off on introducing sweet foods other than pureed fruits until a child is at least a year old. Hold off on nuts and berries till age one.

Calories

When you take away aroma, flavor, texture, and the social aspects of food, you are left with food's rock-bottom purpose—fuel. The food we eat provides the energy we need to keep us going and growing. The energy-producing value of a food is expressed in calories. The federal Daily Recommended Intakes of energy for children are:

- 1,300 calories a day for ages one to three
- 1,800 calories a day for ages four to six
- 2,000 calories a day for ages seven to ten
- After age ten, recommendations vary by gender

Foods high in fat or sugar provide a lot of calories per ounce, but they may be low in nutrients. Nutrient-dense foods like fruits and vegetables are generally lower in calories by comparison, so you can eat more of them for the same number of calories.

Although the three macronutrients—fats, carbohydrates, and protein—can all be used as fuel by the body, each has different qualities. Carbohydrates such as sugars and starches provide quick energy. The more concentrated fats provide sustained energy. Proteins provide the raw materials to build muscle and tissue, but they are used only as last-ditch fuels as they burn less efficiently.

Over the course of a week, roughly 50 percent of your child's intake of calories should come from complex carbohydrates, 20 percent from fats, and 30 percent from protein. Don't obsess about these numbers—just use them as a guideline to help in planning nutritionally balanced meals and snacks. Concentrate on high-quality sources of each of these macronutrients. This is clearly an area for improvement nationally. It's sad but true that American children aged two to eleven get way too many of their daily calories in the form of sodas, "fruit" drinks, and sweet and salty snacks.

Fortunately, it is easy to get all the healthy foods you need with plenty of room for a few treats. Check out our own version of a healthy food pyramid for children. Concentrate on getting the biggest portion of your child's diet from foods and fluids at the bottom of the pyramid. Save the foods at the top for occasional treats. Specific foods listed in each category are examples of the healthiest choices in that food group.

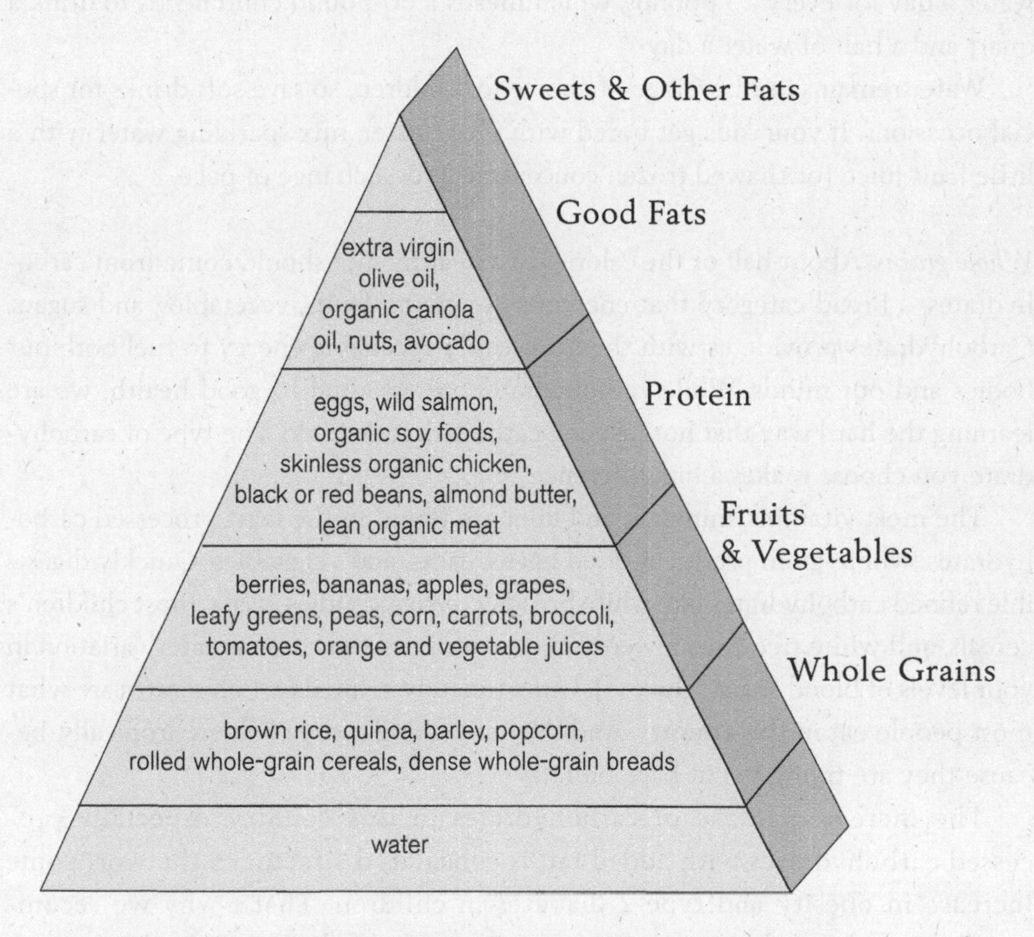

THE HEALTHY CHILD FOOD PYRAMID

Water. Your body may *feel* solid, but more than half of it is water. Your heart, blood, and kidneys must have enough water to filter out and excrete the waste products of the body efficiently. Water also moisturizes the mucous membranes so they can perform their immune duties, lubricates the joints, and keeps the digestive system working smoothly. Yet according to one recent study, 70 percent of preschoolers did not drink *any* water in the course of a day. Children are more vulnerable to dehydration—which can cause dizziness, weakness, constipation, and headaches—because of their smaller size. Children under 80 pounds should drink a cup of water a day for every 10 pounds, which means a 60-pound child needs to drink a quart and a half of water a day.

Water remains our beverage of choice for children, so save soft drinks for special occasions. If your kids get bored with plain water, mix sparkling water with a little fruit juice (or thawed frozen concentrate) for a change of pace.

Whole grains. About half of the calories in a healthy diet should come from carbohydrates, a broad category that encompasses grains, fruits, vegetables, and sugars. Carbohydrates provide us with the most easily accessible energy to fuel both our bodies and our minds. While carbohydrates are essential to good health, we are learning the hard way that not just any carbohydrate will do. The type of carbohydrate you choose makes a big difference.

The most vitamins, minerals, and fiber are found in the least processed carbohydrates: whole-grain products, dried beans, fruits, and vegetables. Quickly digestible refined carbohydrates like white breads, cookies, candies, pasta, most children's cereals, and white rice have fewer of these nutrients and cause greater variation in your levels of blood sugar (glucose). Unfortunately, refined carbohydrates are what most people eat in this country. And they are eating more of them, ironically, because they are trying to cut back on fat.

The increased intake of carbohydrates in this country, especially processed carbohydrates with added fat, is considered a factor in the worrisome increase in obesity and type-2 diabetes in children. That's why we recommend that your children get as many as possible of their carbohydrates from foods like oatmeal, dense whole-grain breads, produce, and whole-grain entrees and side dishes such as barley soup or bean burritos in whole wheat tortillas. Croissant sandwiches, high-sugar cereals, giant cinnamon rolls, and cookies as big as their heads should be reserved for special treats rather than everyday fare.

more on . . .

SERVING SIZE

Servings are so large at many restaurants now that people have lost track of what a normal serving looks like. Keep these amounts in mind whenever you are checking to see how well your kids are meeting their nutritional requirements.

For a preschooler, a serving is: ¾ cup low-fat or nonfat milk, ½ cup yogurt, ¼ cup cooked or ½ cup raw vegetable, ⅓ cup juice, ¼ cup fresh fruit, 1 slice of bread, ¼–½ cup of rice or pasta, 1 to 2 ounces of meat, or ¾ cup unsweetened ready-to-eat cereal.

For a school-aged child, a serving is: 1 cup low-fat or nonfat milk or yogurt, ¼ cup cooked vegetable, ½ cup salad greens, 1 small fruit, ½ cup grapes or berries, ½ cup juice, ¼ cup dried fruit, 1 slice of bread, ½ cup pasta or rice, 2 to 3 ounces meat or fish, ½ cup cooked beans, 2 tablespoons nut butter, 1 egg, or 1 cup ready-to-eat cereal.

The more natural carbohydrates contain healthy insoluble and soluble dietary fiber, which benefits your kids both immediately (by preventing constipation) and in the long-term (by helping prevent cardiovascular disease and diabetes). After the age of two, fiber intake in grams from grains and produce should equal your child's age in years plus five (for instance, 11 g a day for a six-year-old). Unfortunately, only a third to a half of kids between the ages of four and ten meet this standard.

You can help kids meet their fiber needs by keeping ready-to-eat servings of fruits and vegetables in the refrigerator and little bags of almonds or walnuts on the snack shelf for older kids. Learn to cook and enjoy dishes based on legumes like pinto or red beans. Choose whole-grain cereals, and avoid cereals with cartoons on the box. We're floored that manufacturers can strip a grain product of its naturally healthful components, drench it in several forms of sugar, add artificial flavorings and vivid artificial colorings, toss in a few vitamins and minerals, and then maintain that the product is good for your child.

There is some concern that all flours are too easily turned to sugar in the body, but we think banning kid- and lunchbox-friendly foods like bread, tortillas, and pasta would be a nightmare for parents. Make sure that the breads you buy are firm and not squishy, and that they feature whole grains, cracked wheat, or at least whole wheat flour high on the list of ingredients. (Don't be fooled by the term *wheat flour*. It's just white flour.) Most supermarkets now carry gluten-free baked goods and other products for those with celiac disease who have trouble digesting wheat and other grains that contain gluten.

We encourage you to experiment with whole grains beyond whole wheat, oatmeal, and brown rice. Your family might also like quinoa as a side dish, barley in a thick soup, or bulgur (cracked wheat) as the basis of a hot-weather salad. We recommend a few cookbooks to get you started in the Resources section at the back of the book.

Fruits and Vegetables. Children should eat 3 to 5 servings of vegetables a day and 2 to 4 servings of fruit. Study after study has shown the powerful effects of a diet that contains this level of produce. Eating enough fruits and vegetables may help prevent diabetes, obesity, cardiovascular problems, osteoporosis, many cancers, and even some vision problems. These benefits seem to come from the wide variety of antioxidant vitamins and minerals and phytochemicals (plant compounds) found in fruits and vegetables. These phytochemicals, in addition to being antioxidants that neutralize cell-damaging free radicals, also have their own specific effects on our metabolism. The quercetin in citrus fruits, for instance, can reduce the symptoms of allergy, and the lutein in corn and spinach is good for your eyes.

Because there are so many beneficial compounds spread throughout the fruit and vegetable kingdom, our advice is to "eat the rainbow." Eating 5 to 9 servings of variously colored fruits and vegetables a day assures you of getting a full range of vitamins, minerals, fiber, and phytochemicals.

more on . . .

FOOD COLORS

Different colors of fruits and vegetables indicate the presence of different phytochemicals in the plant pigments. Orange foods like squash and carrots tend be higher in carotenes, blue foods like berries tend to be higher in anthocyanins, red foods like tomato are higher in lycopene, and yellow foods like corn have lots of lutein and zeaxanthin.

more on . . .

SAFE FISH

As a source of "good" fats, fish is an important part of a healthy diet, but unfortunately many lake, river, and large saltwater fish also contain environmental pollutants such as pesticides, PCBs, and heavy metals. We recommend feeding children wild Alaskan or canned salmon and other saltwater fish, but not swordfish, king mackerel, tilefish, and shark. Limit tuna to no more than 4 to 6 ounces a week, and choose skipjack tuna over albacore. Check with your local office of the Environmental Protection Agency as to which freshwater fish are safe to eat in your area.

Protein. Protein is essential for growth and development, and it's the basic building block for muscles and tissue. The amino acids that make up each protein molecule are also essential to a whole range of body processes. While young children need about 4 ounces a day of protein, most Americans actually eat far more animal protein than they need, putting a strain on the liver, kidneys, and digestive system.

We don't call this protein category "meat" as so many other charts do, because we would prefer to see folks move toward a more plant-based diet. We put dried beans, nuts, and soy foods into this category in addition to the lean meats and fish usually found there. We don't stress meat because saturated fats from red meat and chicken have been implicated in a host of unhealthy conditions including atherosclerosis (which may start in childhood) and cancer. We are also concerned about additives such as antibiotics, growth hormones, and environmental toxins that are found in most red meat, chicken, and fish. Unless you are able to buy meats raised without antibiotics or hormones, we think that you should limit the amount of red meat and chicken your young child eats, placing a greater emphasis on clean fish and plant-based protein options.

Although it's fine to use small amounts of chicken or fish as flavoring agents, we think it's an even healthier strategy to make legumes, grains, and vegetables the focus of most meals. Try to use more low-fat or nonfat dairy products, soy hot dogs or hamburger (good in vegetarian chili), soy-milk smoothies, bean burritos, and other yummy foods high in protein. Look for organic products when possible, both to reduce exposure to agricultural chemicals and to avoid genetically modified foods.

Dairy. Milk, cheese, yogurt, and other dairy products provide protein, but they are also important sources of the calcium and other minerals kids need to grow strong teeth and bones. Calcium needs vary by age, but range from 500 mg a day for one-year-olds to 1,200 to 1,500 mg a day for ages eleven to eighteen. Although dairy foods are an inexpensive, convenient source of readily available calcium, they are not the only source. Calcium needs can be met by three servings a day of dairy foods or by enough servings from foods such as calcium-fortified orange juice or soy milk, tahini, kale, cooked white beans, and/or supplements.

We have differing opinions about drinking cow's milk. Dr. Russ doesn't believe that dairy foods should be a big part of any child's diet. So while Dr. D's family drinks nonfat pasteurized cow's milk, Dr. Russ's family prefers calcium-enriched organic soy milk. We think all parents should educate themselves on this issue, talk with their pediatricians, and decide what choice is best for their own kids. Whatever your choice, we strongly recommend that you buy organic when possible. Those with lactose intolerance can also buy lactose-free dairy products, or try yogurt and frozen yogurt.

TIP: Consider delaying introduction of milk if there is a family history of allergies, or restricting the amount of milk your child drinks if he or she has had recurrent ear infections, asthma, skin disorders, constipation, or other signs of food intolerance or hypersensitivity. If there is a familial susceptibility to type-1 diabetes, you may decide to avoid cow's milk altogether and get calcium from other sources.

Fats. Fats and sugars are not up there at the top of the food pyramid because they are evil and must be avoided at all costs. We prefer to think of the items at the tip of the pyramid as foods to be eaten—and enjoyed—occasionally. Clearly, fat is an essential part of the diet, and sugar certainly feels like one. But you will get most of the fats you need and more than enough sugar from healthy foods listed elsewhere on the pyramid. This top portion is for the extras like butter, salad dressing, jam, soda, and the full range of empty-calorie snacks.

more on . . .

TEN POWERHOUSE FOODS FOR YOUR KIDS

Optimize your child's nutritional intake by serving foods like these that are packed with vitamins, minerals, fiber, and other healthy compounds:

Rolled oats and other whole grains

Yogurt or milk

Berries

Broccoli and other leafy green vegetables

Soy and other dried beans (soy is also available as milk, soy cheese, meat analogues, etc.)

Wild salmon

Calcium-fortified orange juice

Almonds (chopped or sliced to prevent choking) and almond butter

Tomato

Ground flaxseed

The types of fats and sugars you eat make a big difference to your health. Let's start with fats, which your body needs to provide energy, absorb vitamins, and maintain body heat. The three basic kinds of fats are: saturated, monounsaturated, and polyunsaturated. Most fats and oils are in fact a mixture of all three types of fats, categorized by their predominant form.

- *Monounsaturated fats* from extra-virgin olive oil, expeller-pressed organic canola oil, nuts, and avocados are associated with a reduced risk of cardiovascular disease and some cancers. Most of your child's fat calories should come from foods high in monounsaturated fats.

- *Saturated fats* from meat, dairy products, coconut oil, and palm oil tend to clog the arteries, raise levels of "bad" cholesterol, and increase the risk of certain cancers. Some saturated fats, such as stearic acid (which is converted in the body to the same monounsaturated fat in olive oil), are not harmful, but you should generally keep saturated fat intake low.

- *Polyunsaturated oils* such as corn, soy, sunflower, safflower, and cottonseed oil are unstable oils that oxidize easily and promote inflammation. Limit intake as best possible.

In addition to these three major fats, there are two important fatty acids, one to incorporate in your diet and one to avoid.

Omega-3 fatty acids appear to reduce inflammation, improve cardiovascular health, and elevate mood. These healthy fats are also being studied for their potential to reduce cancer and prevent type-2 diabetes. The modern American diet is low in omega-3 fatty acids, which are found in cold-water fish like salmon and in walnuts and ground flaxseed, so try to include more of these foods in your child's diet.

Trans-fatty acids are artificially created when vegetable oils are solidified in a process called hydrogenation. Partially hydrogenated fats—found in stick margarine and many fried or processed foods—appear to have the one-two punch of both raising bad cholesterol and lowering good cholesterol. The trend is now toward reducing or eliminating trans fats in the diet—New York City actually banned their use by restaurants.

more on . . .

GROUND FLAXSEED

We use a coffee grinder or blender to grind small batches of fresh flaxseeds into meal, and have found that a small, tightly sealed glass jar will keep the meal fresh for a few weeks in the refrigerator. We sprinkle a teaspoon of the nutty-tasting meal on our kids' cereal or salad and add it to smoothies or pancake batter. Just don't use any seeds or meal that smell like paint (a sign of rancidity).

Children under two need fat for proper brain development, so we don't recommend that you try to restrict their fat intake (except for trans fats). After age two, the American Academy of Pediatrics recommends that fat intake gradually decrease so that by age five, total fat over the course of several days averages out to about 20 to 30 percent of calories and is primarily monounsaturated.

Sugars. Sugars are ubiquitous in processed foods. If you read the labels you'll find them not just in the expected baked goods and sweets but also in "fruit" drinks, salad dressings, catsup, and even some spaghetti sauces.

According to federal food surveys, our kids get about 15 to 23 teaspoons of unnecessary sugar every day from soda pop, juice drinks, candy, cakes, cookies, and heavily sweetened cereals. Unfortunately, children who load up on these calorie-rich but nutrient-poor foods don't have the appetite for the good stuff. Soda intake, for instance has a very direct effect on nutrition. Since the 1970s, soda intake by young children has risen 16 percent, while milk intake by young children has decreased by—you guessed it—16 percent. The children consuming the highest percentage of calories from sweets are also the most likely to be getting inadequate amounts of eleven vitamins and minerals, especially calcium. For all these reasons, we try not to even bring soda pop and other sugary foods into our own houses.

Let's face it, human beings like sweet things. But you don't want your children eating so many sweets that they miss out on healthier fare. That's why our first choice for dessert and sweet snacks is whole fruit, which delivers not just natural sugar but a whole range of vitamins, minerals, and fiber. Low-fat, low-sugar fruited and frozen yogurts also fill nutrient needs while satisfying a sweet tooth. Some kids even like to snack on oven-roasted vegetables, especially squash, beets, sweet potatoes, and green beans, which have a natural sweetness missing in vegetables cooked other ways. Let these sorts of high-nutrient-value, flavorful foods be the mainstay of your kids' sweets intake, and you'll be able to cheerfully agree to the occasional soda or ice cream cone.

TIP: To get a better idea of how much sugar is really in a food, look for all the forms in which it may appear–sugar, brown sugar, corn sweeteners, corn syrup, honey, molasses, sorbitol, mannitol, fructose, dextrose, maltose, and sucrose. They all mean "sugar."

more on . . .

DECODING THAT NUTRITION LABEL

Many people make the mistake of just reading the calorie count on a snack food without also checking the serving size and number of servings in the container. As a result, they underestimate the number of calories they're eating and the amounts of fat, salt, and sugar they're taking in. Check to see how closely your version of a serving correlates with the size given on the label. Remember that the amount of fat, sugar, and salt on the label is for one serving, not the whole package.

Even though we have just given you several pages of dietary guidelines, we also want to encourage you to be somewhat relaxed about diet. No child wants to live with the nutrition police. It's far more pleasant, and just as effective, to use more subtle tactics in your campaign to help your family eat better.

- *If you don't want them to eat it, don't bring it into the house.* A lot of food arguments are avoided simply by only having foods in the house that you are willing to have your family eat. Spend an hour at the grocery sometime when the kids aren't with you just reading the labels on all the foods, choosing the brands and varieties that seem healthiest and tastiest. Resolve to buy just those foods in the future. You can throw them in the cart without thinking about it since you've already done the research.
- *If you won't eat it, don't make your kids eat it.* A food or recipe may be very nutritious, but if nobody in the family likes the taste, the pleasure drains out of the meal.
- *Educate your children about foods so they have the information and incentive to eat well on their own.* Then they become the police, not you.

SUMMARY

- Try to incorporate lots of fruits and vegetables and whole-grain foods in your family meals and snacks.
- Rely on monounsaturated fats from olive or canola oils rather than saturated or trans fats.
- Keep healthy options for snacking available and ready to eat.
- Remember, there are no "evil" foods—just foods that should only be eaten occasionally or in small portions.

Our Other Food Concerns

We have a number of scientific, cultural, and political concerns about food that we'd like to touch on briefly. For instance, we think there are good reasons to try to secure clean food and drinking water for your family, but that's a big topic more deeply discussed in chapter 8. We also think it is important to prepare and store foodstuffs safely to prevent food-borne illnesses like *Salmonella* and *E. coli* infections that are becoming more prevalent (and more resistant to antibiotics). This subject is beyond the scope of our book, so we have listed sources of food-safety information in the resources section.

We think there are certain additives used in processed foods that should be avoided. We suggest, for instance, that you avoid the excess sugars and salt often used as cheap filler. In addition to overloading on sugars, the average American child eats 2,948 mg of sodium a day, way over the recommended 1,200–1,500 mg maximum. We also share concerns about some of the preservatives, colorings, and artificial flavorings used in processed foods. For instance, some children are very sensitive to the flavor enhancer monosodium glutamate (MSG), the additive behind the facial tingling of "Chinese-restaurant syndrome." The food dye tartrazine (FD&C Yellow No. 5) may cause itching or hives in some children, and behavioral problems have been linked to it and other food colorings. We also suggest limiting the amount of cured meats, such as hot dogs, that your young children eat, as the nitrites used in curing have been associated in a few studies with the development of some childhood cancers and type-1 diabetes.

In addition to these scientific concerns, we are quite unhappy about the cultural messages our children get about food. First, there is the tremendous commercial pressure on our kids (and therefore on us) to eat unhealthy foods. The shows our children watch are interrupted every few minutes for another snack-food ad, which encourages them to eat even when they are not hungry and to ask for "supersize" meals when they are. Portion size has also been increasing in this country, which raises expectations of what a serving is. In the 1950s, a bottle of Coke held 6 ½ ounces of soda. Now a "child-size" take-out soda is twice that big. And can you remember when cinnamon rolls and muffins weren't as big as the balloons in the Macy's Thanksgiving parade?

In some areas of the country, fast-food franchises pay for the privilege of a spot in the school cafeteria or local hospital, and soft drink giants have contracts for soda machines in school hallways. We find these forms of marketing extremely upsetting both as doctors and as fathers and urge you to speak out against them in your community.

What Parents Can Do

Parents have the power to insure that their children have healthy attitudes about food. No matter what messages the surrounding culture sends, you are the people most able to influence your children by virtue of their love and respect for you. Don't waste this precious capital. If you can gradually integrate some of the following suggestions into your daily life, your whole family will win.

- *Involve your children in all phases of food preparation.* Grow some vegetables on the balcony or plant a garden together. Let the kids pick out new fruits or vegetables to try (star fruit! purple potatoes! yellow tomatoes!). Teach your kids how to cook simple foods and how to prepare the table for meals.

▶ *Become a nutrition educator*. Show them what you can learn from the labels on foods. Explain the standards you apply while choosing food for your family. ("I try to find a cereal that's low in salt and sugar, and ice cream that's low in fat because I love you and want you to be healthy.") Tell little children what's specifically healthy about a certain food. ("Spinach is really good for your eyes.")

▶ *Don't label foods as either "bad" or "good."* Explain that some foods we need to eat often and some foods we need to eat only occasionally.

▶ *Instill and model healthy attitudes toward food as a source of both pleasure and health*. It's OK to go "yummmmm" when you eat!

▶ *Make good food choices easy*. Keep more desirable foods handy in ready-to-eat form.

▶ *Provide a variety of foods*. Don't just focus on one macronutrient or a few standby menus. By eating a wide range of healthy foods your kids will get all the nutrients they need.

▶ *Practice portion control*. Provide your kids with servings appropriate for their size, age, and caloric needs. Use small plates, but let them know that additional helpings are available if they're still hungry.

▶ *Don't skip breakfast*. And don't let your kids skip breakfast, either. The morning brain requires food—preferably carbohydrates—to get kick-started. Kids who don't eat breakfast don't do as well in school. For children, breakfast is also a major source of fiber, vitamins, and minerals.

▶ *Make meals pleasant occasions for the whole family*. Establish meaningful rituals (saying grace, turning off the phone, sharing the high points of the day) that build family closeness.

FAQs about Nutrition

How do you get a kid to eat more vegetables and fruits?

The first trick is to make fruits and vegetables more interesting. Involve your children in the entire culinary process, from planting the seed to growing and serving the food. Kids think it's a lot more fun to graze on snap peas in the garden or pluck a cherry tomato off the pot on the porch than to eat whatever green or yellow thing you stick on their plate.

Then be adventurous with foods. Enjoy trips to the nearest farmers' market or specialty food store, where there are often free samples to tempt kids into trying new tastes.

And finally, make a variety of fruits and vegetables available at all times. Put little bags of dried fruits in an easy-to-reach cupboard and cut-up vegetables in the refrigerator. Keep a filled fruit basket on the kitchen counter. Try the stealth strategy of adding fruits and vegetables to other foods (grated carrots in the spaghetti sauce, zucchini slices on the pizza, cucumbers and tomatoes in the sandwiches, blueberries in the pancakes).

I've got a picky eater. How can I make sure she eats a balanced diet?

Let's start with a new division of labor. It's your job to be a good role model for healthy eating and to serve a nutritious meal or snack. It's your child's role to eat what she wants from it. This avoids a whole lot of arguing over food. Offer a variety of healthy foods, including small amounts of new ones, and insist that she try at least a taste of each. Don't worry if she doesn't seem to eat much at certain stages of growth or if she only seems to eat one thing. Food jags are common in young kids. Save what she doesn't finish for later, and keep healthy snacks such as produce, yogurt, and whole wheat bagels on hand as well. Studies find that children have to encounter a new food eight or more times before they will willingly eat it—it takes time to get used to a new taste or texture—so persevere.

Is fruit juice a healthy drink for my child?

We don't recommend fruit juice in the first year of life as it may cause a child to develop a preference for sweet liquids that will reduce his intake of healthier beverages like water. We don't recommend apple juice for toddlers because it is high in a poorly absorbed sugar called sorbitol that often causes loose stools and abdominal pain. Children who drink more than 12 ounces of juice a day in the first two years of life may lose their appetite for more nutrient-dense solid foods and grow poorly. Those who drink too much calorie-dense fruit juice at later ages are more likely to be overweight. An excess of sweet drinks can also lead to more dental cavities, too. In our opinion, moderate amounts of diluted grape juice or orange juice are better fruit-juice options for older children, especially those with a tendency toward obesity.

My four-year-old never clears his plate without a battle. What can I do?

Maybe you're overestimating what he can eat. Preschoolers aren't generally big eaters. Just offer a few tablespoons each of a variety of foods and ask him to take at least one bite of everything on his plate as "an adventure." Children will naturally eat as much as they need. Do not force an unwilling eater to clean his plate. You want your child to learn how to tell when he is hungry and when he is not, and eat accordingly.

What vitamins, minerals, or other supplements should I give my child?

We'd much rather children got all their essential vitamins and minerals from food, but we are realistic enough to recognize that this isn't always possible. A good children's multivitamin is clearly no substitute for proper nutrition, but it is a way to hedge your bets. Look for a product that contains a range of vitamins and minerals. While there is no set rule regarding amounts of supplemental vitamins and minerals for children, a five-year-old should probably not be taking more than 50 percent of the adult Daily Recommended Intake of most vitamins and minerals.

We both recommend a daily multivitamin and an omega-3 supplement (200 mg/day for toddlers, 400 to 600 mg/day for ages four to seven, and 600 to 800 mg/day for kids aged eight and up), with the addition of a probiotic containing at least

10 billion CFU for kids with allergic issues, frequent infections, or frequent courses of antibiotics. Dr. D recommends calcium and often an iron supplement too. Dr. Russ advises vitamin D for all children and calcium only for preteen and adolescent girls.

More is not necessarily better when it comes to vitamins, especially the fat-soluble vitamins A, D, E, and K, which can be toxic in high doses. We have both seen children whose skin has turned orange from too much vitamin A. A child can get several times the recommended daily intake of A for his age from the combination of his multivitamin and boxed juice drinks containing the adult DRI for the vitamin. Be sure to factor in all sources of supplementation. For safety's sake, keep all child and adult supplements where children absolutely cannot reach them. Children commonly overdose on vitamins, which is especially dangerous in the case of those containing iron.

How do I handle my child's sweet tooth?

Use the power you have as the only people in the house with a debit card and a driver's license to regulate what foods are available there. If you don't bring it into the house, it can't be eaten there. Occasional sweets are fine as a treat, but don't make a habit of stocking them.

Are some sweeteners better than others?

The debate continues about the potential adverse effects of artificial sweeteners, and even though there is no proven evidence of harm, we prefer to err on the side of caution. People with an inherited metabolic disorder known as PKU (phenylketonuria) clearly cannot use aspartame (Nutrasweet), and too much sorbitol, a sugar alcohol often used in sugarless gums and candies, can cause diarrhea in children. We are more concerned about long-term effects of chemical sweeteners, which is why we advise the use of natural sweeteners when needed—sugar, real maple syrup, honey, or an herb called stevia that can be found in health food stores (1 or 2 drops should give you the sweetness you desire). Be aware, though, that raw honey should not be given to children under the age of two because of the risk of infant botulism, a very serious illness.

What oils are best for my family?

Look for oils that are liquid at room temperature. Avoid as many partially hydrogenated oils as possible. The oils with the best fat profiles are high in monounsaturated fats and low in saturated fat. In order of monounsaturated content, the top oils are hazelnut, extra-virgin olive (our favorite), high-oleic-acid safflower oil (not regular safflower oil), avocado, almond, canola, mustard, and walnut.

My daughter is a vegetarian. How can I make sure she gets the nutrients she needs?

Children can thrive on vegetarian diets if they receive enough calories and care is taken to make up for essential nutrients such as vitamin B-12, iron, zinc, calcium, and vitamin D that are normally derived from meat, eggs, and dairy products. Without these nutrients, vegetarian children are at risk for poor growth, anemia, and deficiency diseases. Vegan children (who don't eat any animal products) have to be even more careful about including alternative sources of micronutrients than do lacto-ovo-vegetarian children (who eat dairy and eggs but no meat). Parents of vegetarians should provide a wide variety of grains, legumes, and organic soy foods to make sure their children get all the essential amino acids. Concentrated sources of calories like nuts, seeds, soy foods, avocados, and dried fruits can help insure they get enough calories as well. Consider a daily multiple vitamin and mineral supplement as well as a safety net.

What are some healthy snacks for kids?

There's no end to the healthy snacks available for kids. For example, there's almond butter on a whole wheat bagel, peeled baby carrots, air-popped popcorn (try it with nutritional yeast sprinkled on top), hummus on a warm pita bread, low-fat organic string cheese, frozen grapes, fruit-juice popsicles, yogurt, cut-up vegetables with a low-fat dip, fruit smoothies of organic soy or regular milk blended with organic strawberries and/or a banana, squares of organic soy cheese or a soy hot dog, a handful of almonds or walnuts, and dried blueberries—be creative. You'll find some helpful guides listed in the resources section of this book.

CHAPTER 6

Don't Just Sit There:

Exercise and Physical Fitness

Many American children are busy from dawn to dusk. They jump from bed to the school bus, spend five or six hours sitting in the classroom, come home for a few hours in front of the TV or on the computer with their friends, lie on the floor doing homework, and finally, protesting their lack of sleepiness, stagger off to bed. Once a week religious instruction, music lessons, sports practice—or all three—might be squeezed into the schedule. Our kids' lives are so jam-packed it's no wonder that we parents don't even notice that one essential factor for their good health is often missing.

This missing element—we'll call it Factor X—has amazing powers. It can sharpen the mind, reduce anxiety and depression, build energy, reduce weight, increase immune function, improve sleep, increase strength and flexibility, and lower the lifetime risk for diabetes, heart disease, osteoporosis, Alzheimer's disease, and certain cancers. If we told you a nutritional supplement delivered all these benefits, you know you would jump at the chance to buy it for your family. And if we told you it was free? That remedy would be flying off the shelves.

So how do you get Factor X? You move. Factor X is exercise. People underrate the value of exercise, but remaining physically active throughout the day is an unbeatable strategy for good physical and mental health. And it's cheap. You really don't need much more than a pair of walking shoes, a jump rope, or a favorite dance tape to get all the exercise you and your kids need for next to nothing.

But, you ask, don't kids already get plenty of exercise? Aren't they busy all the time with all sorts of activities? Don't they get phys ed at school? Despite all their apparent busyness, our kids are just not moving their bodies around enough every day. Unlike children from earlier generations, they spend less time in vigorous outdoor play or physical chores. They don't walk or ride their bikes to school or the store. Too many are couch potatoes, immersed in fascinating but sedentary activities. This inactivity is a prime factor in what experts call "an epidemic of obesity" in American children. Sadly, obesity is now the number one childhood disease in America, and our children are on the way to becoming the fattest generation of adults in American history, with all the health problems that implies. Doctors who treat children now not only have to deal with the usual childhood health problems, but they must also help protect their young patients from taking the first steps toward serious health conditions in adulthood.

Maintaining a Healthy Weight

Before we continue with the topic of physical activity, we'd like to talk a little about the problem of obesity. This topic fits perfectly between our discussions of nutrition and exercise, because obesity is caused by the interplay between food intake and physical activity. Although genetics plays a part in childhood obesity, the reason American children are increasingly overweight boils down to two things—they eat too much of the wrong foods and they sit around too much.

Overweight is generally defined in one of two ways—as a measure of body composition called the body mass index, or BMI (calculated by dividing weight in pounds by the square of height in inches), or as a percentile that refers to the child's weight for height compared to other children of the same age. Children are generally considered at risk for being overweight if their BMI is between the 85th and 95th percentile of weight for height on a growth chart. Being in the 95th percentile of weight for height signals that the child is already overweight, a condition that is likely to persist into adulthood unless changes are made. Keep in mind, however, that there are more variables to the BMI in children, whose actual percentages of fat-to-lean mass may vary by gender, race, stage of development, fitness, height, and sexual maturity. The BMI chart in your doctor's office is a guideline only.

How bad is the problem? According to national health surveys taken at regular intervals since the sixties, the number of overweight children in America has increased dramatically, especially in the past twenty years. About a third of children aged six to nineteen are now overweight, and about 11 million of them are obese. Children of certain ethnic minority groups—Native Americans, African Americans, Hispanic Americans, and Asian Americans (especially Pacific Islanders)—are more likely to be obese.

However, the obesity epidemic can't be blamed on genes. Human genes haven't changed as much in the past 20 years as body weight has. Besides, genetically susceptible children (and adults) who eat well and stay physically active can keep their weight within normal bounds. The obesity that appears to run in families may just reflect the passing down from parents to children of poor habits of health, fitness, and nutrition. (New research suggests that exposure in the womb to high levels of blood sugar may turn on genes associated with appetite and weight in the developing child that may then be passed on to the next generation—yet another reason for pregnant women to make good lifestyle choices.)

The five factors most often blamed for the epidemic of childhood chubbiness:

1. *Inactivity*. Toddlers in less-than-ideal day care situations may spend much of the day plunked in front of a TV show or video rather than doing the important developmental work of crawling, walking, tumbling, and otherwise honing gross motor skills. Older kids don't seem as interested in good old-fashioned play—running, jumping, climbing trees, or making up active games—as they are in sedentary amusements. The greatest obesity is seen in the children watching the boob tube most.

2. *Advertising*. When was the last time you saw an ad for a fruit or a vegetable on kids' programming? There's a food ad every five minutes during Saturday-morning cartoons. No wonder our kids are always grabbing us by the sleeve in the grocery store and begging for some sugar- and/or fat-filled food product.

3. *Not eating together*. Kids get an increasing number of their calories away from home, and when they are eating at home, there is often no adult with them to make sure they are eating well.

4. *Higher-calorie drinks*. Kids, especially overweight ones, may get a lot of their daily calories from sugar-filled juice drinks, sodas, and energy drinks. Kids who down two or three of these a day may be getting 20 to 30 teaspoons of sugar and killing their appetite for more nutritional foods.

5. *Fewer high-fiber foods*. Kids are eating fewer of the low-calorie, high-nutrient carbohydrates like fruits, vegetables, and whole grains, and more products made of white flour, sugar, and unhealthy fats. There is some evidence that fiber plays an important role in weight control.

Is chubbiness really so bad? At certain stages in their development—in infancy, or just before (boys) or during (girls) puberty—children naturally tend to be a little chubbier. But weight gain at other times should be a warning. For instance, children are meant to be lean from after the age of one until about age five or six, when they begin to put on weight again. This turning point around age five is called the point of adiposity rebound. New research suggests that kids whose adiposity rebound occurs too early, because they aren't encouraged to be active or because they overeat, are at double the risk to become obese adults.

Obesity is linked to a scary array of childhood health problems, including asthma and allergy, type-2 diabetes, high cholesterol, fatty liver disease, and high blood pressure. It's also a cause of social problems such as bullying. Overweight children who become overweight adults are at greater risk for such conditions as gall bladder disease, kidney disease, breast cancer, and colon cancer. Public health experts worry that the current increase in obesity will lead to greater disease and disability as adults, possibly shortening the average American lifespan by as much as five years. It's clear to us that keeping your children fit is a great way to protect their health now and in the future.

more on . . .

TYPE-2 DIABETES

Of particular concern is the dramatic rise in type-2 (non-insulin-dependent) diabetes in children, especially minority children. Unlike the autoimmune, insulin-dependent form of diabetes that is known to occur specifically in children, type-2 diabetes was unheard of in kids until very recently. Often called adult-onset diabetes, it was considered solely a problem of the old and sedentary. The appearance of type-2 diabetes in children is particularly alarming, because the disease progresses more rapidly in kids, and it puts them at higher risk for all the complications of diabetes—atherosclerosis, hypertension, kidney failure, blindness, and impaired circulation—at an earlier age.

How to Help an Overweight Child

We don't want you (or your child) to obsess unnecessarily about her or his weight—there's enough obsession with weight and body image in our society already. But we do want you to take your pediatrician or family practitioner seriously if he tells you that your child is heavier than average for his or her height. Parents are often the last to realize that their children are overweight. If other culprits, such as endocrine disorders, have been ruled out, use this warning flag as a signal to do an evaluation of your family's nutritional intake and energy expenditure. It could be you've let some good habits slip and merely have to reinstitute them. Or you might need to begin to make a few changes to move your family toward a healthier lifestyle. The most effective programs for child obesity do not single out the overweight child. Instead they try to instill healthier behaviors in the entire family—starting with the parents.

Preventing Obesity

Since childhood obesity is easier to prevent than it is to cure, we recommend you follow these tips for all children, even those of "normal" weight:

▶ *Take a good look at yourself.* Of children who are overweight, 80 percent have parents who are overweight. Parental influences—for good or ill—are decisive, because the dietary and activity patterns set in childhood tend to be permanent. Be prepared to make changes in your own behaviors to become a good role model. You might even want to turn the tables and ask your kids to give you stars or stickers for exercising more, or making better food choices!

▶ *Breast-feed your child.* Even just a few months of breast-feeding lowers a child's risk of obesity up to 40 percent.

▶ *Teach your child how to tell when she is hungry.* Learning to recognize the sensations of hunger and satiety may help a child avoid the kind of mindless eating that causes excess weight. Teach your children to "check in" with themselves when reaching for a snack and ask, "Am I really hungry, or do I just need a glass of water or something else to do?" Respect natural hunger instincts and don't force young children to finish everything on their plates. Remember, it's your job to put healthy food on the plate, it's their job to decide what and how much to eat.

▶ *Get more active.* Start small and work up to a total of 45 minutes of exercise, all at once or scattered through the day. Once again, don't underestimate the power of your own example on your children. If you take a positive approach toward movement, they will too. Even the mundane calorie-burning household physical chores—sweeping, washing the car, vacuuming—can be made to seem like fun.

▶ *Limit TV, video, and computer time.* Kids in America spend more time watching one screen or another than they do at any other activity except sleeping. And the more hours they spend there, the more likely they are to be obese. Unless you're willing to hook a stationary bike up to the TV and make your kids work for their screen time, we suggest you limit free-time use of TV, video, or computer and keep those screens in areas of the house where you can monitor their use.

IS YOUR CHILD AT RISK FOR OBESITY?

Here's a quick and easy test of your child's risk for obesity:

1. Give yourself one point for each time your child eats fast food in a week (write zero if none).

2. Add one point for each soft drink (pop, juice, juice drink, energy drink) your child drinks in a day.

3. Add one point for every time your child eats candy, dessert, ice cream, cookies, or other sweet/salty treats in a day.

4. Add one point for every hour a day your child spends sitting in front of a computer/video/TV screen.

5. Take away one point for every fifteen minutes your child is vigorously active during the day.

6. Add one point for each parent who is overweight or obese.

Total your score. If it adds up to six or less, you're doing well. If the score ranges from seven to eleven, start making gradual improvements in nutrition and activity levels. If the score is twelve or over, you need to start work right away on the areas with the highest scores.

▶ *Stress quality foods.* Overweight children might not eat a greater *volume* of food than normal-weight children, but their choices are often higher in empty calories from added fat and sugar. Use casual conversations while buying, preparing, or eating food together to educate your child as to which foods are for every day and which are for once in a while.

▶ *Make sure there are always "everyday" foods available in the house and in the car.* Always provide low-calorie, high-impact foods like carrot sticks, nonfat yogurt, and apples.

▶ *Eat meals together*. When you sit down together at the table, you gain more control over what your children eat and improve everyone's chances for a nutritionally complete meal.

▶ *Grow a backbone*. Don't give in to big-eyed pleas for the latest high-sugar cereal with a TV character on the box, high-fat Lunchables, nearly juiceless "juice drinks," and the darling little individual bags of candies and snacks that "everybody else has." An occasional treat is fine, but your message about better choices in food should be a consistent one.

▶ *Think about serving size*. In this world of "supersize it," people have lost sight of what constitutes a single serving. Toddlers, for instance, only need several tablespoons of a variety of foods, not big, heaping servings.

▶ *Make water the beverage of choice*. Overweight children especially get too many calories from sodas and fruit drinks.

▶ *Tuck them in earlier*. Insufficient sleep appears to be related to weight gain. Be sure to put your children to bed each night at a time that permits them at least eight to ten hours of sleep.

▶ *Teach stress management*. Stress, in and of itself, increases the potential for weight gain by increasing cortisol levels, impacting metabolism, and negatively affecting sleep patterns. Some people also turn to food when under stress. (For more on stress management, see chapter 10.)

Never Say "Diet"

We don't believe that parents should make kids diet. Growing children—even overweight ones—need enough energy and nutrients for development, so any reduction in calories to lose weight should really only be a small one. Instead of talking about weight loss, we talk to kids about weight maintenance, encouraging overweight kids to stay at the same weight as they grow taller until they reach a healthier weight-to-height ratio. We put the focus on making better food choices rather than restricting intake, and on increasing the number of calories burned in physical activity.

Fitness is really the goal here, not thinness. This is an important distinction, because our culture tends to equate thinness with acceptability—a terrible lesson for a child. The weight-maintenance approach allows children to monitor their own height and weight and feel good about themselves and their bodies. It also decreases the chances of tipping a child—especially a girl—into an eating disorder or depression.

Obesity should be treated as a family issue. Research suggests that obesity in children is difficult to control unless the whole family is involved. Don't single out the overweight child for special treatment—everyone in the family should be eating well and exercising. In fact, a recent study found that obese kids lost more weight when the program focused on the parents as agents of change than when it focused on the overweight child.

The Exercise Prescription

It may sound flip, but exercise, in one form or another, really is good for whatever ails you or your kids—and it's fun too. It can improve conditions as varied as obesity, high cholesterol, depression, stress, back pain, and even fatigue. It can give a kid a real boost of energy when she feels like her tail is dragging. In fact, Dr. D has been known to require teenaged patients with mononucleosis to walk to his office for their visits because he knows how much more quickly they will recover with a little exercise. Exercise can also help prevent such chronic conditions as diabetes, osteoporosis, hypertension, and atherosclerosis—all of which can have their roots in childhood.

We believe strongly in encouraging children to be physically active, for both the immediate benefits of exercise and the long-term health protection it provides. Parents are key players in this effort, because 95 percent of kids who are physically active have parents who are too. You're not an athlete? No problem. You only need to be active. You don't need to be good. It's the effort that counts more than the results. Besides, we're convinced that there's a sport or activity for every taste and talent. Your preference could be walking or dancing, lifting weights or swinging a tennis racket, riding a bike or pushing a lawnmower at top speed. Pick whatever's fun. Those who require variety might even do a little of everything.

TIP: Take advantage of technology. Kids may be more willing to walk or get on the exercise bike if they're hooked up to a radio or an MP3 player, and more willing to move if there's one of those new active "exergames" on the Wii or the game player.

When we use the word "exercise," we don't mean boot-camp calisthenics or 26-mile marathons. We just mean physical activity. Walking around the neighborhood, shooting a few hoops, working in the garden, rolling around on the lawn with the dog, washing the car, jumping rope, dancing to your favorite CD, playing hide-and-seek or Sardines, tossing a Frisbee or a baseball. None of these activities require planning or expense—just get up and get going.

Yet we don't do it. And, as a consequence, our kids don't either. Three out of four kids are not getting enough regular activity to protect their current and long-term health. Our children get less active with age, especially girls, who by the time they are ten are getting only half the exercise they did when they were six. Girls who are active are able to build the strong bones they will need to protect them through life, and they may be reducing their risk of breast cancer in adulthood as well.

The Importance of Play

American kids spend less time in simple, unstructured, child-directed play because they're busy staring at a screen, playing organized sports, or taking after-school lessons. But play is important for child development. Play is children's work—more fun than our own perhaps, but just as vital. Play is the way young children educate their bodies and minds and exercise their creativity. Free play—unorganized and uncontrolled by adults—gives them a chance to develop and refine their motor skills, learn about the world, become aware of how their bodies move through space, learn to get along with others, learn to amuse themselves, and use their imaginations. When you plunk a young child in front of a TV or video for too long, you stop this process and encourage passivity.

Young children love to move around, so your principal role in the early years is not to discourage them. Allow them to be free of restraint as much as is safely possible, out of their strollers and playpens and into the world. Sure, it's more trouble for you, but it's very good for them. As they get older, you can help them find activities that are fun for them and encourage them to try all sorts of exercise, from tumbling to team sports to dance and movement. They may only be able to handle short sessions of ten minutes or so at first, but kids age five to twelve should be getting at least thirty minutes a day of physical activity of various types. There is some evidence that forcing children to exercise backfires, producing adults who refuse to move a muscle. So rather than shoving a recalcitrant child onto the playing field, you may be better off focusing on more indirect strategies: finding activities that interest your child, rewarding increased activity, providing more active family experiences, and being a positive role model yourself.

What Kind of Exercise is Best for Children?

You want cardiovascular exercise as well as activities to build strength and flexibility. Children need weight-bearing, high-impact activity too—such as tumbling, dance, or jumping rope—to build bone mass during this crucial period. We feel strongly that for safety's sake, all children should also learn to swim. We advise you to include some form of all three of the major forms of exercise in your family activities. For instance:

1. *Aerobic exercise*. Aerobic exercise, sometimes called cardiovascular exercise, works the heart and lungs as well as the muscles. The goal is to raise your heart rate, increase oxygen intake, and improve stamina. Running, swimming, soccer, basketball, bicycling, aerobic dance, and brisk walking are all forms of vigorous aerobic exercise. So is playing a family game of run-and-chase. We both squeeze lots of aerobic activity into our children's lives in little daily bits and in longer weekend outings.

2. *Strength training*. Strength training, or resistance exercise, increases muscle strength and endurance by working a muscle against resistance in the form of weights, elastic tubing, or a person's own body weight. Generally a certain number of repetitions ("reps") of an exercise are done at a certain weight, gradually moving on to heavier weights or more repetitions as the exercise becomes easier. Methods include Nautilus-style machines,

exercises with stretch bands, push-ups and pull-ups, and weightlifting with dumbbells. Young children can get resistance exercise most easily by doing exercises like modified push-ups that use their own bodies as the weight. Well-supervised teens can use free weights or machines if they stick to light weights and more reps.

3. *Flexibility exercise*. Stretching exercises and yoga stretch muscles, tendons, and ligaments to improve flexibility and balance.

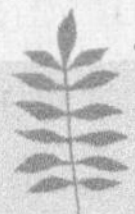

TIP: Be sure to teach your children to warm up with gentle exercises, jogging in place, or stretches before any extended period of vigorous exercise and to cool down in the same manner after the session.

In addition to different forms of exercise, there are different intensities as well. For instance, the activities of daily life—strolling to the car, climbing stairs, taking out the garbage—are generally considered to be light exercise. Walking and other activities that expend calories without working up much of a lather are considered moderate activities. In contrast, running or circuit training—exercise that makes you sweat and boosts your heart and breathing rates—is considered vigorous. All three intensities of activity are beneficial. More intense workouts provide more benefit, but the fact remains that any exercise is better than none. Once you and your family make the big decision to become more active, you can start small and gradually work up to more active time as everyone starts to experience how good it feels to move around more.

Kids and Sports

We think that children should stick with free play until age five or six. After that age, you can start them in more structured community sports programs whenever their motor skills and cognitive skills are ready for the activity and the teamwork. This timing is very individual. Just because the neighbor's child is ready, don't assume yours is. As a parent, make sure the focus during the elementary school years is on learning basic skills (how to kick or hit a ball) and on fun, not competition. The fun part is important. Of the 20 million kids who start organized sports, 6 million drop out by age thirteen. Those who drop out are often sports-loving kids with limited to moderate skills who end up spending too much time on the bench or feel too much pressure from coaches and parents when the emphasis shifts from having fun to winning at any cost.

We're strong supporters of team sports when started at the right age and with the right attitude, because sports were very important to both of us growing up. We have encouraged our kids to continue school and league sports as they get older. Aside from keeping kids fit for at least a season, these sports programs teach fair play and provide an opportunity for social interaction, the experience of teamwork, a chance for mentoring by a caring adult, a sense of belonging, and an identity ("I'm a runner"). If you're lucky, the kids will be too busy with sports to get into trouble, and the habit of exercise may carry over into adulthood.

The Importance of Physical Education

Walk into any school that features the new PE, and you'll regret every minute you ever spent waiting in line to toss the ball in the basket during your own school years. These kids are all active, engaged, and having fun. The first graders are in a huge circle stretched along the perimeter of a huge rainbow-colored parachute. They raise it together and in waves, lower it, dance under it and back out again, run clockwise and counterclockwise, laughing and gazing in delight at the billowing cloth. Older kids jump rope, double dutch, in a display of fancy footwork you can only dream of emulating, before moving on to juggling—an impressive show of hand-to-eye coordination. In other classes kids enjoy everything from folk dancing to traditional sports like basketball and soccer, but with a difference—everybody plays.

This is the kind of physical education we want for our kids. The tide is turning against programs that keep kids on the bench or waiting in line for half the period, that focus only on competitive team sports, that drill for outmoded physical fitness tests, that separate kids into the "cans" and "cannots," that seem more like boot camps than fun. We are big fans of the new PE because it puts the emphasis on personal fitness rather than competitive sports, with the goal of acquiring lifelong skills and habits of exercise. This change for the better is coming not a minute too soon.

Despite the Department of Health and Human Services Healthy People 2010 goal of increasing both the number of students getting PE daily and the amount of time they are actually active in those PE classes, very few states meet recommendations for 30 minutes of PE a day for elementary students and 45 minutes a day for middle-school students.

PE is being squeezed out of the core curriculum for a number of reasons: the belief that physical exercise is a "frill," the lack of financial resources in strapped school districts, and a lack of time as more and more required topics are added to the academic program. But parents need to speak up to school administrators and school boards about the value of PE. Good PE classes encourage healthy behaviors that benefit our children now and save society health dollars in the future. PE helps protect our children from cardiovascular and other chronic disease, controls weight, teaches teamwork, improves sleep, builds self-esteem and feelings of competence, relieves stress, and passes on the idea of fair play. Physical education classes provide a safe place to exercise, an important issue in some areas where the parks and playgrounds may be unsafe for kids, and they provide access to equipment and venues that families may otherwise not be able to afford. Daily PE even appears to help with academic learning.

We list some resources for parents in the back of the book, but you should know how to evaluate your children's PE program. In our opinion, there are ten things that a good PE program should do:

1. Occur daily for 30–45 minutes, depending on grade level

2. Offer a variety of age-appropriate and enjoyable activities that spur the learning of basic motor and social skills

3. Focus on cardiovascular fitness, flexibility, agility, and muscle strength rather than on specific sports

4. Keep students moving for most of the class period, with both warm-up and cool-down periods

5. Focus on cooperative rather than competitive games (no losers)

6. Teach skills and activities that foster lifelong fitness

7. Include different types of activities over a period of time so kids with different abilities and interests get a chance to shine

8. Partner with parents through ideas for family activities, periodic individual reports, or parent fitness nights at the school

9. Promote healthy nutritional and exercise behaviors outside of class

10. Be fun—do the kids and teacher look happy?

Let's Take a Break

In addition to organized physical education classes, elementary school kids need breaks for movement during the school day. The precious 15 to 20 minutes of running-around time morning and afternoon that we call recess is the only thing that makes sitting in class all day bearable for many kids. Yet, responding to a push for stronger academics and new federal testing requirements, about 40 percent of school districts across the country have eliminated recess or are considering doing so. We can't understand why parents aren't up in arms about it. Adult workers get coffee breaks. Even the Marines get hourly breaks in their training. So why should we expect our children to do without a refreshing break?

We think eliminating recess undercuts public health campaigns promoting activity and flies in the face of all the developmental research on the importance of play to learning. An integrative approach to education requires not just educating the mind with academics, but also the soul with the arts, and the body with PE and recess. Recess helps kids burn off excess energy, increases alertness, stimulates brain development, exercises their imaginations, and improves their socialization skills. In fact, we think there's a possible connection between the loss of opportunities for activity in the school day and the increasing use of medications for problems of inattention.

If your children's elementary schools are cutting back on recess, we urge you to work with teachers and school administrators to bring it back. Maybe parents can volunteer to help oversee playgrounds during these breaks. We include some recess-preservation resources at the back of the book.

Keeping Your Kids Active

Add more activity to your own day. Children admire and want to emulate their parents. What lessons do you want to teach them?

Make some family time active time. Why not play a game of catch after work or bike together on the weekend? Or teach kids some of the simple outdoor games you used to play, like Red Rover, Capture the Flag, Duck Duck Goose, Simon Says, Running Bases, and Sardines. You'll help your kids, and yourself too.

Limit TV/video/computer time. The American Academy of Pediatrics suggests none for kids under two, and no more than one or two hours a day for older children. We go further, and advise just 30 to 60 minutes of free-time screen time on a weekday. Toss away the remote controls and make them walk over to change the channels.

Discover what kinds of physical activities your kids enjoy. Kids who are forced into sports or activities they don't like may be turned off exercise for life. Attend games as often as you can, practice with them, offer positive feedback, and make sure that the experience remains fun and not a source of stress for your child.

Encourage children to walk more. If safety is an issue, walk with them. You'll get both a little exercise and a little extra time together.

Ask your kids what they do in PE class. If it doesn't sound like enough, observe a class. If necessary, lobby with teachers, principals, and your school board for a better program.

Make sure your kids stay hydrated when they exercise. Thanks to sports bottles, drinking water throughout the day can become as automatic a habit for your children as clicking on their seat belts.

Assign your children chores that keep them moving. Dusting, vacuuming, weeding, and taking out the compost or the garbage all count as exercise.

Avoid labeling your children as "athletic" or "unathletic." Many kids who are considered unathletic at age eight or nine do quite well in sports later. Concentrate on making sure they are fit and happy, because a foundation of fitness will allow late bloomers to reach their peak potential.

Get involved in community efforts to increase the number of parks, playgrounds, recreation centers, bike lanes, walking trails, and playing fields available for the children in your town or neighborhood.

Think ahead. Commit yourself to keeping your children fit to protect them from adult problems like osteoporosis, diabetes, and atherosclerosis that have their roots in childhood.

CHAPTER 7

Just Sit There:

The Importance of Rest and Relaxation

Ah, the bliss of a stolen afternoon at the ball game, an evening laughing with friends, a walk along the beach, or even a few minutes of peace and quiet in the shower. These moments of relaxation are essential for our physical and emotional well-being, no matter how fulfilling our lives. Taking time to play or rest nourishes the soul and helps us cope with the stresses and strains of daily living.

Right about now you're probably thinking, "Relax? Who has time to relax?" You're juggling jobs, chores, and parenting duties while trying to maintain all the personal relationships that are important to you. If you're a single parent, you are beyond busy. There aren't enough hours in the day to do all that has to get done, and we're asking you to take time off to do . . . nothing? Yes, that's exactly what we're doing, and we're doing it with the full knowledge that we don't always practice what we preach.

Parents and Stress

Even though this is a book about your children's health, we are going to take a moment to focus on you parents first, because we cannot tell you how to protect your children from the physical effects of stress without addressing the role of stress in your own lives. Like obesity, anxiety is often a family affair. Our kids absorb a lot of anxiety from us. Although we like to think that we are protecting them from our adult worries, they can sense tension in us and respond with anxiety of their own. If you've ever doubted that parents transfer their stress to their children, just work in a doctor's office for a week. We know from experience that nothing will soothe an anxious child until the parents' worries are addressed and the big folks relax. We have actually seen children with inflammatory bowel disease begin to suffer less pain and fewer bouts of diarrhea after their *parents* have been taught breathing exercises and other stress-reduction techniques.

Once you recognize the two-way flow of anxiety, anger, and other stress-related emotions between parents and kids, you can start learning how to modify your responses and make the whole family healthier. For instance, learning how to control your anger (a big risk factor for heart attack in adults) not only improves your own health, but offers a healthier model for your children as well.

The life of a parent is full of demands on our time, energy, patience, and compassion. We are sleep deprived and always on call. As the enforcers of unpopular decisions, we may get no respect. We postpone our own needs and desires to insure that we are present for our kids, and we often feel inadequate as we juggle our responsibilities and try to do everything as well as we did before we had kids. You couldn't come up with a better recipe for stress!

Every parent feels stressed at some time or another, especially stay-at-home moms and dads. We encourage people struggling with the pressures of raising children to seek out parent support groups, parenting classes, or family therapy—places where they can talk freely without fear of being labeled a bad parent. Don't be afraid to ask for help when you need it.

How Stress Affects Us Physically

As integrative doctors, we know that mind and spirit have incredible effects on the body—for good or ill. Just as physical problems can affect your mental state, your thoughts and emotions can affect the workings of your body. (See chapter 10.) If you are always tired, irritable, and overwhelmed by your responsibilities, eventually your body will pay the price. In our experience, stress is often ignored as a contributing factor to illness. This is partly because of the negative connotations of the term *stress-related illness*. Most people hear the phrase and think, "The doctor is telling me it's not a real illness, that it's all in my head. Everyone will think I'm weak or faking it if I don't have a physical reason for all this pain."

We've seen people who are so unwilling to accept the fact that stressful situations may be affecting their children's health (or their own) that they'd rather push for more tests and more advanced medications than look more closely at their own lives. We have had parents stalk angrily out of the office at the suggestion that something in a child's home or school environment may be creating or worsening a physical problem. This is a shame, because it is far more effective to treat the root cause of a chronic illness than its symptoms, far kinder to try the gentler approaches before the more invasive ones, and far less expensive to try to deal with possible factors like stress before diving into a sea of diagnostic testing. Parental insistence on "medicalizing" what may be a stress-related response reinforces the child's role as a sick person and makes it that much harder to uncover and deal with the emotional issues triggering the problem.

Let's face facts. Everyone has stress. It's how you deal with it that matters. Admitting to stress is not a sign of weakness or personal failure. Denying stress does not make it go away. We have to learn how to recognize stress in ourselves and how to defuse it before it does damage. When stress is chronic, or when it is not well managed, we suffer from side effects, such as neck and back pain, digestive problems, anxiety and depression, and headaches. One theory is that our subconscious mind resorts to provoking physical discomfort to get our attention when we repress unwelcome emotions. These pains are a signal that we need to take the time to deal with an issue we are trying to ignore. A pain in the back or the neck provides a legitimate excuse to slow down. We like this theory because we have seen for ourselves how often muscular or stomach pains disappear once their real causes are understood and addressed.

In children, stress is associated with a wide range of problems, including feeding difficulties, colic, frequent colds, diarrhea, bed-wetting, abdominal pain, cough, headaches, motor tics, and wheezing attacks. Young children are especially vulnerable to the effects of long-term exposure to stress hormones, which can slow down growth, brain development, and sexual maturation. Adolescents whose immunity is lowered by the pressure of academic demands show up frequently in our offices with recurrent infections of all varieties, especially during the dark months of winter.

more on . . .

SETTING YOUR CHILD'S STRESS THERMOSTAT

There's increasing belief that our stress thermostats—the regulatory mechanisms that decide how quickly and how intensely we react to stress—are set in the earliest years of life. A child who grows up in a household with trauma, abuse, or lack of parental care and concern may be more emotionally reactive and carry a more negative bias throughout life. A child who grows up in a warm and loving family whose parents foster a positive attitude toward life is more likely to have the resilience to cope well with life's slings and arrows later.

It's not just the acute crises in life—illness, death of a loved one, divorce, moving—that cause trouble. The cumulative effect of the little stresses of daily life—the reactivity to all of life's petty frustrations from losing a toy to a misunderstanding with a friend—can create physical distress too. Learning how to manage the big and little stresses in their lives is one of the greatest gifts for good health you can give your kids.

Learning to Relax

The *relaxation response* is the name given to the cascade of physiological reactions that returns the body to normal after it's been in a fight-or-flight state. By decreasing heart rate, blood pressure, and muscular tension and producing a feeling of deep relaxation, regular practice of techniques that evoke the relaxation response can minimize and even resolve physical symptoms. In addition, classroom training in stress reduction has been found to improve learning, improve grades, reduce tardiness and absenteeism, increase self-esteem, and reduce aggressive behavior.

There are many ways to trigger the relaxation response, among them meditation or prayer, breath work, biofeedback, hypnosis, guided imagery, and progressive muscle relaxation. We'll discuss the specifics of these relaxation techniques in the chapter on mind/body medicine, but the box on the next page lists five quickies that can be used any time and any place.

FIVE MINI-RELAXATION EXERCISES

Breathing exercises like these are believed to release neurotransmitters that promote relaxation.

1. *Atten-SHUN!* Close your eyes and focus your attention on your breathing. Is it fast? Slow? Ragged? Strained? Try to make it as slow and regular and relaxed and easy as you can.

2. *Backwards count.* Close your eyes and exhale. As you inhale, say the number 2 to yourself; as you exhale, say the number 1. Continue slowly and evenly, focusing your attention on the flow of air through your nose or mouth and your counting.

3. *Balloon breath.* Imagine there is an empty balloon in your lower abdomen and let it fill and empty in three stages. First breathe deeply in, gently filling the balloon so that your belly slowly pooches out. Keep breathing and let the upper part of the balloon expand so your ribs expand out to the sides. Fill the very top of the balloon, so that your breastbone slowly rises toward your chin. As you exhale, reverse the process. Let the air out of the top of the balloon so the breastbone sinks, then bring the ribs back in, and finally deflate the balloon in your belly.

4. *The 4-7-8 breath.* Rest the tip of your tongue on the ridge of tissue above the inside surface of your upper front teeth, and keep it there throughout the exercise. Close your mouth and breathe in through your nose for a count of four. Hold the breath gently for a count of seven. Open your mouth and release the breath with an audible whoosh over a count of eight. Repeat for a set of four. At first, you may have to speed through the count to get to seven before you run out of breath, but with practice you'll be able to count more slowly.

5. *Nosing around.* Take deep breaths in through your nose and slowly out through your nose.

Children and Stress

You may not believe that children can suffer from stress, but it's true. In addition to the stress in their own lives—standing at the free-throw line in a close game, giving an oral report, trying to be cool—our kids also absorb anxiety from us. We like to think they aren't aware of the big issues we are dealing with—problems in our marriage, financial tension, job insecurity, substance abuse—but they sense it all and are sometimes more stressed because they do not have the experience or the full information to quiet their fears.

Children have to deal with the same anxieties about living up to expectations that we all have. And many parents and schools have set the bar high, pressuring their children to succeed in all things. Family therapists now see elementary schoolchildren with chronic stress-related headaches, stomachaches, and free-floating anxiety from parental pressure to excel. It's no wonder that about 30 to 40 percent of the sick children we see are there for conditions caused or worsened by stress. The sources of stress and the way it is expressed may differ, but both adults and children should always be open to the possibility that stress is involved in medical and behavioral problems.

We often say that the pediatrician's office is where parents trying to hide stress from their kids meet kids trying to hide stress from their parents. Children sometimes internalize stress to protect their parents. If doctor and parent are willing to consider the possibility that stress is a factor, a child's physical problem may become the spark that sets off parent-child discussion of other issues previously unnoticed or repressed.

CLUES YOUR CHILD IS STRESSED

Children may exhibit the same signs of stress as adults–nervousness, muscle tension, irritability, depression, fear, headaches, sleep disorders, and neck, back, or abdominal pain. Children also have symptoms of their own. A child who is whiny, clingy, fearful, withdrawn, staggered by even minor change, or hyperactive may be stressed. A child who is suddenly stuttering, wetting the bed, sucking his thumb, acting out, or changing his eating habits may be stressed. A child suffering from recurrent colds or sinus infections–signs of a depressed immune system–may be stressed.

The top three stress-related conditions we see are abdominal pain, headache, and cough. Many parents are quite familiar with "school-day tummy" and tension headache, but few realize that chronic cough can have an emotional component as well. Dr. D also sees lots of thirteen-year-old boys with what he calls "Bar Mitzvah syndrome." In the weeks and days before this important and stressful religious ceremony, many of them come to see him with headaches, abdominal pain, and acute infections. Once he explains the role of stress, however, symptoms ease up. After the ceremony, they disappear.

Always look for a physical cause for your child's symptoms first. If no organic cause is found, don't assume that the symptoms themselves are not real. The pain your child feels from, say, a stress-related abdominal problem, is as real as that of appendicitis. The child is not faking the pain. The pain may be caused or worsened by stress, but it is still real, and parents should treat it as such. Some parents are unable to accept the idea that their child would sense and respond to stress in so physical a manner. Others resist the mind/body approach because they think it implies their child has a mental problem. In fact these stress responses are quite normal and show an awareness of one's circumstances and environment. Once mom and dad accept this diagnosis, parents and physicians can help the child understand that these symptoms are actually coping mechanisms, and everyone can work together to discover the root of the problem.

If you suspect your child is stressed, there are several things you can do:

- Examine the stresses in your own life and consider how they might be affecting your child.
- Take steps to bring your own stress under control.
- Talk to your child in an open-ended way about things that might be bothering her.
- Explain what stress is (see box on the next page), and help her identify any stress reactions she may be having.
- Brainstorm ways to relieve this stress. Teach her coping skills or relaxation techniques to use in stressful situations. (See chapter 10.)

more on . . .

EXPLAINING STRESS TO YOUR CHILD

Once a child understands that her symptoms are an attempt to cope with stressful thoughts or events, she can begin to alleviate them. We start by explaining what stress is and how it differs from fear or excitement, which share some of the same physical signs. We remind a child how stepping up to the plate with the bases loaded, riding on a thrilling roller coaster, or sitting down to a pop quiz can make our hearts beat faster, our palms sweat, our muscles tighten, and butterflies jump around in our stomachs. Stress causes the same symptoms and more, because it's a nervous feeling with no place to go, and they disappear once the test, the solo performance, or the roller-coaster ride is over. But the stress of unspoken thoughts and fears can cause physical problems that last until these secret concerns are eased. Sometimes we don't talk about them because we are ashamed or afraid. Sometimes we are not even aware of our worries until our bodies send us a wake-up call.

If physical symptoms persist, make an appointment with her pediatrician or family practitioner to discuss them. Be wary if your child's doctor suggests psychotropic drugs such as antianxiety agents, "muscle relaxers," or sleeping pills. Too many doctors and parents appear more willing to give children drugs for their own convenience rather than taking the time to identify and address the emotional root of the problem. But both hyperactivity and depression can be symptoms of stress in children. We strongly urge you not to jump into medicalizing what may well be a stress-related problem.

De-Stressing Your Family

It's not easy to find time or space to relax. In fact, it's probably been hard to find the time to read this book! So once again, our advice is to be kind to yourselves and just do what you can. A good first step is just learning that there are things you can do to relieve stress. Trying to make one stress-reducing change in your life is a good second one. We're betting that once you've learned the power of a mini-meditation or a moment of prayer to modulate your reaction to stress, you'll be motivated to try a few more of these ideas. We hope eventually you will come to realize that stress management is as important to health as exercise and good nutrition.

- *Learn a relaxation technique and use it regularly*. (See chapter 10.) As the old saying goes, "If Mama (or Papa) ain't happy, ain't nobody happy." Then teach your kids a few simple tools to manage stress and explore with them the times they might be useful. Describe body cues they can use to monitor their stress levels.

- *Give your kids the emotional vocabulary to explain and understand their feelings*. Get the older ones journals where they can vent and explore these feelings.

- *Practice saying no to more than you can handle*. Put a family calendar of activities in a prominent place, and make sure no one is overscheduled. This may require limiting the number of activities each child does in the course of the school year. Be sure to leave open spaces in the schedule—everyone needs free time to dream, to reflect, to make art, or to play a musical instrument. If everyone in the family seems to be speeding around unnecessarily, try to slow the pace.

- *Spend at least some time one-on-one with each child every day so you can catch little worries before they become big stressors*. Squeeze in a little time for a one-on-one with yourself, too—even if it's only fifteen minutes in the shower.

- *Sit down for family meals together as often as possible*. Turn off all cell phones and PDAs during the meal. The entrée can be pizza, but take the time to light some candles and express your gratitude to set the tone.

- *Limit TV/video/computer time to an hour a day, especially on school days*. These forms of entertainment/education are generally fast paced and high adrenaline, so avoid them close to bedtime. Be tough about the media that your children are allowed to see.

- *Establish relaxing rituals that are meaningful to you*. It may be prayer at certain times of the day or a family stroll after dinner. Relaxing bedtime rituals like reading aloud, playing soft music, receiving a brief massage, or reviewing the gifts of the day can help kids (and their parents!) unwind.

▶ *Avoid caffeine and sugar*. Frankly we cannot understand why parents would even consider offering their children caffeine-laced soft drinks such as Pepsi, Coke, and Mountain Dew, but they do.

▶ *Make sure everyone gets enough sleep*. Kids need between nine and fourteen hours of sleep a day, depending on age. Many of us live in constant sleep debt, which is not good for either physical or mental health. (See chapter 23.)

▶ *Be mindful of your world*. There's beauty all around us, if we only look for it. Try doing just one thing at a time so you can give it your full, unstressed attention.

▶ *Laugh more*. When the tension level in your family is mounting, do something to help blow off steam—a funny walk contest, a pillow fight, or a goofy movie. Your kids will have a good time and the child in you will get a chance to be silly for a while.

more on . . .

THE RESTFUL HOME

Ideally your home should feel like a sanctuary from all the rush and pressure of the outside world. Unfortunately, at least one study has found that kids' cortisol levels–a good measure of stress–are actually much higher at home than at school. There are many ways to make the family home a more restful place. You might use colors in the house that make you feel happy or soothed; instead of all white walls, consider peach, soft blue, sage green, golden yellow. Experiment with scents that you find relaxing. Lavender, sandalwood, lemon, rose, vanilla, and apple are usually considered sedative. Reduce the clutter in your house and you'll reduce both the frustration when you cannot find anything and the wearing sense of continual disorder. Try silence or some soft music at certain times. Bring in more flowers, plants, or other signs of the natural world. Get a pet. If you live in a noisy place, think about buying a white-noise machine or a pleasantly gurgling indoor fountain. Set up one area–even if it's small–where family members can go for peace and quiet. Make it comfortable for reading or noodling around with arts or crafts. Remind your family of all the people who love them by displaying photos of grandparents, aunts, uncles, cousins, and special friends around the house.

CHAPTER 8

It's Not Just What They Breathe:

Protecting Your Children from Environmental Hazards

When you hear the words *environmental threat*, do you think of oil spills or chemical leaks? If so, you're seeing only part of the picture. In this chapter we'll be focusing on risks to your children's safety in their immediate physical environment—the places where they live, play, and study. Your children's health may be affected not only by chemicals on the lawn or pesticides on the food, but also by their failure to use a seat belt or a bicycle helmet.

As integrative physicians, we've seen the many ways a child's physical environment can affect health. We've treated children born with fetal-alcohol syndrome (FAS) and extremely low-birth-weight babies born to heavy smokers. We've treated children with abdominal pains, seizures, learning disabilities, and mental retardation from exposure to lead; children gassed by carbon monoxide from an inadequately vented heater; children whose asthma gets worse every time the air pollution index is up; children poisoned by household cleaning products.

We'll be talking here about what we think are the greatest environmental threats to your children and what you can do about them. Our aim is not to make you throw up your hands in despair. We just want to give you the information and the tools to protect your kids—and yourselves. Our major areas of concern are the personal safety of children and the safety of the food they eat, the water they drink, and the air they breathe. We leave it to you to determine your own priorities among these issues and how best to act on them. Because we don't have room to go into depth on any of these topics, we are including a list of helpful organizations, books, and Web sites in the resource section at the back of the book.

The Big Picture

You may be tempted to skip this section. After all, you just want to know how to keep your kids healthy. But unfortunately, the health of the environment strongly influences the health of the people who live in it. You can make sure your kids eat right and exercise, but if the water they drink is tainted with chemicals, or if the air they breathe is too high in ozone or full of toxic particles, your best efforts will be undermined. Your children are indeed what they eat—and what they breathe and drink, as well. While our primary concerns may be with our own children and our own neighborhoods, we urge you to think and act more broadly so that everyone benefits.

A great deal of environmental progress has been made since the first Earth Day teach-ins in 1970. So are we done yet? Unfortunately, no. Although many of our past environmental messes have been cleaned up, others linger, even fifty or sixty years later. DDT and other toxic chemicals banned years ago are still so pervasive that they can be found in the tissues of nearly every human on Earth. In addition to these old environmental insults, we are drowning in a sea of chemicals, combined in an endless number of ways in new products, whose long-term effects are unknown. These toxic substances so far have been linked to miscarriages, infertility, neurological disorders, developmental problems, cancers, birth defects, intellectual deficits, behavior disorders, and respiratory illness. So, yes, there's still work to do.

Our children are exposed to toxins and carcinogens daily. Yet our society still places more value on economics—the right to sell chemical products of uncertain safety or the cost of cleaning up brain-damaging lead from old housing stock—than on our children's health. Consider the fact that there are seventy thousand synthetic chemicals registered with the Environmental Protection Agency (EPA) that can be sold and used even though less than 20 percent of them have been assessed for their potential to harm children—who are uniquely vulnerable to their effects. Consider that we know that exposure to lead in old house paint severely impacts young children, yet we don't make lead abatement a budget priority.

If you think about it, it is surprising that our safety standards for nearly all environmental toxins are based on adult exposures. After all, pound for pound, children take in more air, more food, and more water—and whatever contaminants they contain—than do adults. They have different (and sometimes weaker) mechanisms for getting rid of toxins, and they absorb toxic elements (such as lead) at proportionately higher rates than do adults. Not only are they exposed to more toxins, but they are at greater risk of an adverse response to them as well. Their little bodies are in a constant state of development in which major growth and maturation may be triggered or stunted by the slightest hormonal or nutritional nudge. It is well known that toxic exposure has more long-lasting effects the earlier in life it is sustained, and that exposures during key periods of development are more likely to be irreversible.

Exposures Before Birth

Exposure to the environment begins even before a child meets the world firsthand. There is a growing body of evidence that toxic damage can occur before birth and even before conception through damage to eggs and/or sperm. That's why we recommend that all adults of childbearing age follow on-the-job safety procedures and limit their exposure to toxic metals and chemicals as much as possible. Pregnant women should be especially careful of the new life developing within them. The fetus is exquisitely sensitive to chemical and toxic influences because its cells are dividing, differentiating, and growing so rapidly.

Alcohol and tobacco smoke—two common substances we do not normally think of as environmental pollutants—readily cross the placenta to cause developmental and physical damage such as physical abnormalities and learning and behavioral problems. Low levels of lead, mercury, or certain chemicals transmitted by the mother can also affect the future child's intellect and development, while higher levels have been suggested to play a role in the development of antisocial—even criminal—behavior. The brain is especially vulnerable in these early stages of development because the blood/brain barrier—the protective shield that restricts toxins in the blood from gaining access to the central nervous system—is not fully functional until six months after birth. There are also concerns that hormonally active agents (HAAs) such as pesticides, dioxins, and polychlorinated biphenyls (PCBs) may cause reproductive, nervous, or immune-system problems in the developing children exposed to them. Several studies have found these chemicals in the amniotic fluid of pregnant women.

It is not clear how many of these pollutants are passed to an infant through mother's milk. The average woman's breast milk does usually contain the pesticides, dioxin, and PCBs so ubiquitous in the environment that they are considered "background" contamination. Experts agree, however, that it is far better to breast-feed than not to breast-feed. Human milk contains so many valuable compounds that breast-feeding still provides a net benefit (except in cases where the mother is on certain medications toxic to the infant or has a transmissible viral illness such as HIV).

more on . . .

WHY KIDS ARE MORE VULNERABLE

▶ *Size.* They breathe more air, eat more food, and drink more water per pound of body weight than adults.

▶ *Food choices.* They eat a smaller variety of foods, increasing their exposure to the specific pesticides and other chemicals used on those crops.

▶ *Activities.* Children live closer to the ground, where they breathe in or absorb through their skin solvents and pesticides in carpets, lawn chemicals, and household dust. They suck their thumbs, bite their nails, and put everything in their mouths, including old paint chips and other soil contaminants. They also play outside more, where they are exposed to particulates and ozone.

▶ *Developmental stage.* Rapidly developing brain and nervous systems are more susceptible to damage. Environmental toxins may interfere with the development of organ systems, which are normally triggered by very subtle variations in natural hormones at very specific times.

▶ *Defenses.* Infants and children absorb toxins more easily and are less able to get rid of them.

We believe that we must put the health and development of our children first and find the funding and the will to protect them from environmental pollutants. We agree with Dr. Phillip Landrigan, head of the Center for Children's Health and the Environment at Mt. Sinai Hospital in New York City, who wrote, "By default we are conducting a massive toxicological experiment in the United States, and our children are the experimental animals."

We've divided the environmental pollutants that most concern us into three categories: heavy metals, organic solvents, and pesticides. We would like to explain a little about the dangers of each, how your child is exposed to them, and what you can do to reduce their exposure. We haven't room to touch upon any of these issues in great depth, so remember to check the resources section at the back of the book for other sources of information.

Heavy Metals

Mercury

This is the toxic metal that concerns us the most. While we worry that mercury-amalgam dental fillings may pose an unnecessary health risk, we are much more concerned about mercury pollution from other sources. Mercury compounds released into the air from coal-fired power plants and waste incinerators drift down to pollute soil and the water. Aside from the immediate risk to neighbors of these plants, the greatest exposure may come through eating large predatory fish at the top of the food chain whose fat contains concentrations of the toxic metal from smaller fish they have eaten. Other potential sources of exposure: broken mercury thermometers, illegal dumps, and certain folk medicines and charms, especially from the Caribbean.

Exposure to mercury compounds can lead to neurological deficits, and there is an increasingly large body of research tying mercury exposure to autism. While there were some concerns about the ethyl mercury in vaccines preserved with thimerosal, studies have found that even after the removal of mercury from nearly all vaccines given to children, autism cases have *increased*, not decreased. The focus has now turned to methyl mercury from environmental exposures, so it is all the more essential that we get the mercury out of the air we breathe, the soil we play on, and the fish we eat.

more on . . .

MERCURY AMALGAM FILLINGS

There exist enough theoretical concerns over mercury-based dental fillings that we recommend against their use for new cavities. However, most experts believe it better to leave existing mercury amalgams in place until regular wear and tear requires them to be replaced. Their removal may actually release more mercury into one's system through both blood and vaporized material.

Lead

Lead poisoning has decreased dramatically since the metal was eliminated from gasoline and paint in the 1970s, but the American Academy of Pediatrics estimates that one in four kids under six years of age still has significant exposure to lead. How are our kids exposed? Mostly through dust, dirt, and water. In older neighborhoods and near heavily trafficked roads, lead from car exhaust from years past and fine particles of pre-1978 lead-based house paint have been deposited in the soil over the years. Dust formed by the opening and closing of windows with old layers of lead paint on them is another major source. Lead can also be found in drinking water that travels through old lead water pipes and faucets, and even from the fumes from candles with lead wicks. Anti-lead campaigns are usually aimed at protecting poor children living in dilapidated housing, but more affluent parents remodeling older homes are now discovering that their children may be at risk as well.

The neurological consequences of lead poisoning can be great: lowered IQ, learning disabilities, hyperactivity, aggressiveness, and criminal behavior. A two-to-three-point loss of IQ has been associated with every 10 mcg/dL (micrograms per deciliter) increase in blood-lead level. We know that developing embryos are more likely to have poor developmental outcomes if their mothers have elevated levels of lead in their blood (often from lead stored in their bones since their own childhood and released into the blood during pregnancy). Early exposure to lead appears actually to shrink areas of the brain associated with attention, decision-making, and emotional control—especially in young males.

The optimal level for lead in the blood is zero. Federal safe blood-lead levels are set at 10 mcg/dL, though it's known that damage occurs at even lower levels. Reducing our children's exposure to lead will be an expensive undertaking that may require government subsidy, but it must be done or we risk damaging innumerable children.

Nine Ways to Protect Your Children from Heavy Metals

1. *Buy an easy-to-use testing kit with wipes that turn color in the presence of lead, especially if you live in an older home*. If lead levels are elevated, follow lead-abatement measures such as replacing old windows, sheet-rocking over painted surfaces, and hauling away tainted soil. Move out during any remodeling and have the house carefully cleaned after the work is done. Wipe down walls and other surfaces regularly with a damp cloth to remove lead-laced dust. Take off shoes before entering the house to reduce the amount of dust tracked in. Wash toys frequently, especially those that end up in your child's mouth. And don't buy toys that may contain lead.

2. *Have your child's blood-lead levels checked*. We recommend having your child's blood tested for lead at ten to twelve months and again at two years if you suspect your house or soil might contain lead. Also test any newly adopted children from other countries. If tests are normal, you and your doctor can decide whether to continue with annual tests. If not, the first step is to identify the source of exposure and remove it. In severe cases, detoxification therapy (chelation) may be recommended.

3. *Make sure your children eat foods rich in calcium and iron*. Low levels of these minerals appear to speed the uptake of lead. Pregnant women need adequate levels of calcium (1,000 to 1,300 mg a day), so lead is not drawn from their bones into the blood supply they share with the fetus.

4. *Test your household water for lead using an inexpensive screening kit*. If the pipes appear to be the problem—and they are accessible—replace them. Otherwise, get a water filter that not only removes lead but also addresses any other pollutants in your water.

5. *Dispose of thermometers, batteries, compact fluorescent light bulbs, and all other sources of heavy metals properly as hazardous waste.*

6. *Request lead checks of the schools, day care facilities, community centers, and other buildings where your children spend time.*

7. *Avoid fish.* The usual recommendation is for pregnant women to avoid eating big ocean-going carnivorous fish like swordfish, king mackerel, tilefish, and shark, or fish from local lakes and rivers, as these fish may contain high levels of mercury or other toxic metals. We think it's better to be safe than sorry, and so we ask pregnant and nursing women not to eat any fish at all and to get their omega-3 fatty acids through a purified fish oil supplement instead. Children and nursing women should limit how often they eat those big saltwater fish, as well as albacore tuna. (Skipjack tuna is a better choice.) Check the state-by-state freshwater fish warnings listed at www.epa.gov.

8. *Do not give your children patent remedies from China, India, Mexico, or the Caribbean.* Folk medicines containing heavy doses of lead, mercury, and other toxic metals are responsible for up to 30 percent of all cases of childhood lead poisoning.

9. *Be cautious with candles.* Some candle wicks use lead as a stiffener. When they burn, they may put enough lead into the air to exceed your child's safe daily lead intake! Look for candles guaranteed to be lead free, and don't overdo their use in tightly closed rooms.

Organic Solvents

Solvents are used in the production of many household products. The volatile compounds found in gasoline, dry-cleaned clothes, home-cleaning products, chlorinated water, plastics, carpets, plywood, and many other everyday products are especially dangerous because they evaporate at room temperature and so are easily absorbed by inhalation, skin contact, or ingestion. Organic solvents (most of which are volatile organic compounds or VOCs) are often to blame for what is called "sick-building syndrome."

more on . . .

ENDOCRINE DISRUPTORS

Solvents like chlorine combine with organic materials in the environment to create a large family of hazardous chlorine by-products. Among them are dioxin and other organochlorines, which are all hormonally active agents (HAAs). Called endocrine disruptors or environmental estrogens, HAAs have the ability to mimic or interfere with the normal actions of human hormones that determine how a body develops and functions. In wildlife–and in laboratory testing–HAAs have been associated with such long-term effects as motor delays, behavioral problems, learning disabilities, cancer, breathing problems, decreased reproduction, gender abnormalities, and precocious puberty. It seems likely that HAAs have their greatest effects on the developing fetus or the very young child, stages when the body is very sensitive to hormonal cues in developing the major body systems.

Exposure by either parents or children to organic solvents has been linked to a number of health problems including infertility, miscarriage, birth defects, low birth weight, and childhood cancers. For instance, studies show a connection between a father's on-the-job exposure to industrial solvents and brain tumors in his children. Perchlorethylene (PCE) and other solvents used in dry cleaning not only cause miscarriage in pregnant women but also are rapidly expressed in the breast milk of nursing mothers. Despite the dangers of these volatile compounds, the most worrisome organic solvent is still alcohol. Drinking alcohol during pregnancy can cause serious lifetime defects in the yet-to-be-born child.

High levels of the chlorine compounds created in the process of disinfecting drinking water have been linked to a number of health risks, including certain cancers. We don't want to eliminate chlorination of water—it's essential to protect us from water-borne diseases such as cholera—but we do think you would be wise to filter your water or let it sit overnight in the refrigerator to give the volatile compounds a chance to dissipate. Putting a filter on the showerhead is very important too. A ten-minute shower provides more exposure (via skin and lungs) to chlorine by-products than you get from drinking two quarts of the same water. Make sure your shower filter is a type that works well with hot water. Pregnant women should be especially careful, as excessive exposure to chlorine by-products has been linked to a higher rate of stillbirths.

Nine Ways to Protect Your Children from Organic Solvents

1. *Don't drink alcohol while pregnant.* As far as we're concerned, this is non-negotiable.

2. *Don't smoke tobacco in the house.* In addition to carbon monoxide, nicotine, and carcinogenic tars, cigarette smoke contains solvents like formaldehyde. Children who live with adults who smoke indoors have higher rates of respiratory illness and ear infections, decreases in lung function, and greater risk for sudden infant death syndrome.

3. *Be careful with plastics.* HAAs such as phthalates and bisphenol-A (BPA) are often used to make plastics harder or softer. When you microwave foods in plastic wrap or plastic containers, these chemicals can migrate into your lunch. Make sure baby bottles are made of glass or plastic free of these compounds. The same recommendations hold for the ubiquitous plastic water bottle. We don't recommend reusing single-use plastic water bottles. But if you must, use one with #5 on the bottom, and hand- rather than machine-wash it. Better yet, recycle that old bottle and get one made of stainless steel.

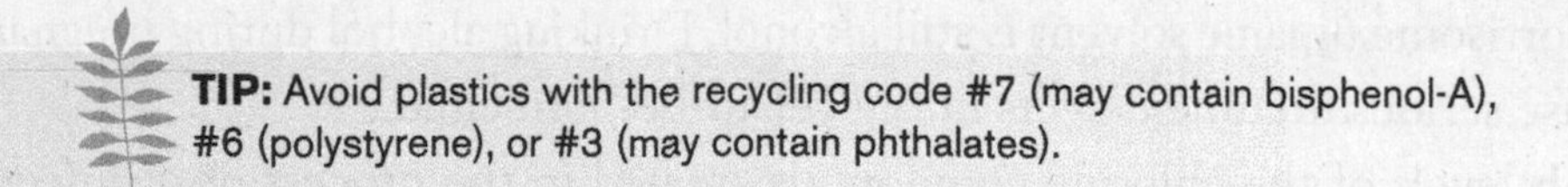

TIP: Avoid plastics with the recycling code #7 (may contain bisphenol-A), #6 (polystyrene), or #3 (may contain phthalates).

4. *Buy nontoxic carpets, paint, and other remodeling materials that don't contain volatile organic compounds.* Be cautious with arts and crafts supplies used by your children too—especially markers and airplane and instant glues—which should be used under supervision and in well-ventilated areas.

5. *Use nontoxic citrus or vinegar-based cleaners in the home.* Limit your use of chemical cleaning products, disinfectants, and room deodorizers.

6. *Install a filter on your faucets and showerhead to reduce exposure to chlorine by-products.* Use a home-testing system or a water-testing company to identify the specific types of pollutants that might be present in your drinking water, and then install the water-filter system that best removes those specific compounds.

7. *Remove the plastic covering on all dry-cleaned items and hang them outside or in the garage until they lose their chemical smell.* Better yet, find a cleaner that doesn't use solvents. And we hereby excuse all pregnant women from picking up the dry cleaning.

8. *Be careful about rubber duckies.* Make sure your children's bath toys, squeeze toys, and teethers are guaranteed free of the phthalates DEHP and DINP, hormone-disrupting chemicals commonly used in the soft rubbery toys that kids love to chew.

9. *Don't allow your children to pump gas for you.* We suggest using the automatic-fill lever and keeping everyone inside the car while the gas is pumping into your tank.

Pesticides

We use the term *pesticides* to mean all synthetic chemicals that kill insects, weeds, fungi, nematodes, and rodents. Pesticides concern us not just because trace residues permeate our foods but also because they contaminate the water we drink and the soil we walk on. We already have a certain level of constant exposure to the most persistent of these chemicals, but we would like to protect our children from any additional exposure.

There is clear evidence that pesticides lower immune function, increase the risk of some cancers, and cause neurological and developmental problems in those with the most direct exposure to them. In agricultural areas, where exposure to pesticides begins before birth and continues through childhood, pesticides have been linked to such problems as memory deficits, decreased stamina and motor ability, autism, and slowed intellectual development, as well as Parkinson's disease later in life.

Although there is less research on the long-term effects of the lower doses of pesticides to which most of us are exposed, it's not a huge stretch of the imagination to think that agricultural chemicals designed to poison, destroy reproductive capacity, damage nervous systems, and disrupt endocrine systems of pests might affect humans adversely too, especially young ones whose various systems are still developing.

We are very concerned that allowable pesticide residue standards do not yet include enough protection for pregnant women and for children. Government agencies are now required to consider the special vulnerability of children while setting safe pesticide levels, consider all possible routes of exposure (and not just food), and take into account the possible synergistic behavior of exposure to multiple chemicals (as generally happens in the real world). This process, however, is moving very, very slowly—largely due to budget constraints.

We don't want to scare you so much about pesticides that you cut back on the fruits, vegetables, and whole grains your children need. These foods contain a wide range of known and as-yet-unidentified compounds necessary for good health. Some of these compounds can even help balance out any potentially harmful effects from pesticide exposure. But we do urge you to consider making a few changes in your shopping and eating patterns to reduce your child's exposure. For instance, you should always wash your produce or buy certified organic produce when possible.

TIP: Washing your produce with a solution of one part white vinegar to three parts water removes many pesticides and kills 98 percent of the germs. Keep the solution in a spray bottle, spray enough to coat the surface of the fruit or vegetable, and rinse with cold water.

If you can't afford to buy organic produce all the time, decide whether you can grow some yourself, buy organic for younger children who are still developing, or just buy organic versions of the foods your children eat most. Remember, children eat a lot more of some foods than adults do, and so have increased exposures to any contaminants on or in them. That's why we are more concerned about the seven to nine pesticides used (and left) on apples, for instance. The typical one- or two-year-old child drinks thirty times more apple juice, eats thirteen times more applesauce, and eats five times more apples (relative to body weight) than the typical adult. If your children consume a lot of apples in one form or another, you can either offer a fruit known to have fewer pesticide residues or make the commitment to buy only organic apple products.

Just knowing which fruits and vegetables are the most likely to carry a heavy burden of pesticides is a good start. The Environmental Working Group (EWG) regularly publicizes a list of the "dirty dozen" and their "cleaner" alternatives. (See box below and our resources section.) The EWG says that such substitutions can halve your exposure to pesticides.

THE FRUITS AND VEGETABLES WITH THE MOST AND LEAST PESTICIDES

The Dirty Dozen (starting with the worst):	**The Cleanest Twelve (starting with the best):**
Peaches	Onions
Apples	Avocados
Sweet bell peppers	Frozen corn
Celery	Pineapples
Nectarines	Mangoes
Strawberries	Frozen peas
Cherries	Asparagus
Lettuce	Kiwis
Imported grapes	Bananas
Pears	Cabbage
Spinach	Broccoli
Potatoes	Eggplant

Our children are also exposed to pesticides through chemicals used at home, in school, and in parks. These are areas where parental involvement can make a huge difference. Pesticides and herbicides are routinely used in many school districts to control insect and animal pests, maintain athletic fields, or beautify the landscape. In some cities and states, school officials are already required to use less-toxic alternatives when available or to notify parents before use.

Then there's the home. According to the EPA, about 71 million pounds of insecticides, herbicides, and fungicides are used by families in their homes and yards. That means that parents can drastically reduce their children's exposure to pesticides (and the solvents that are also included as "inert" ingredients in many of these products) merely by cutting out home use. There are a few studies linking the use of home pesticides to cancer and neurological disorders in children. Among the resources at the back of the book are several that will help you find safer substitutes for bug sprays, lawn chemicals, flea collars, head-lice shampoos, etc.

Four Ways to Protect Your Children from Pesticides

1. *Have your drinking water tested for pesticides, solvents, and other chemicals, and filter it if necessary.* This is especially relevant if you live in an area that is currently or formerly agricultural. People in new subdivisions built in former fruit orchards, for example, have found high levels of agricultural chemicals in their soil and water. The EPA can tell you how to get your own well tested and how to access testing results for your local water company (often available online).

2. *Peel and/or wash your produce*. You don't need expensive produce washes. Either a short soak in a lot of cold water or a few sprays of vinegar-and-water solution, followed by a rinse in running water, should do the trick.

3. *Buy organic when you can*. Focus on fruits and vegetables like apples or peppers that are usually high in trace residues, or on the kinds of produce your kids eat the most. Substitute "cleaner" crops for "dirtier" ones, say broccoli for spinach, or American grapes for imported ones.

4. *Relax about the lawn*. Switch to organic lawn-care products or let a few dandelions pop up—kids love them.

Safe Drinking Water

Since drinking water can contain any or all of the three classes of pollutants we've been discussing, we're making a special place to talk about it. The quality of drinking water varies dramatically from one community and region to another and from source to source. A typical contaminant in one place might be rare in another, and vice versa. For instance, an agricultural town dependent on groundwater from wells might have problems with nitrates from fertilizers, whereas a more industrial area might find solvents seeping into their drinking water source. Communities that rely on rivers or lakes might be more vulnerable to industrial pollution or biological contaminants like bacteria or viruses. Water that is alkaline, or "soft," might be more likely to leach heavy metals from older plumbing within the house.

Many public systems provide excellent drinking water. You can find out if your provider is one of them by checking the Consumer Confidence Report (CCR) it is required to file with the EPA on a regular basis. (See Resources.) You can check the water for the presence of other questionable compounds through one of the laboratories recommended by the EPA. If you live in an older home, you might also want to check the water that comes out of your own taps to reassure yourself that it is not contaminated with lead. If you have doubts about the quality of the water, investigate and install the home water-filtration system that best addresses the contaminant profile of your water.

Be aware that bottled water is not necessarily better than what comes out of your own faucet. Some of the 4 billion gallons a year sold in bottles is, in fact, just tap water that has been "polished" for better flavor but is not necessarily pure.

Think Globally, Act Locally

If you're feeling depressed about the enormity of our environmental problems, remind yourself how far we have come in environmental consciousness, education, and action in the past thirty years. Impassioned individuals and environmental groups have helped make everyone more aware of the connection between environmental health and human health, and brought many important issues into the mainstream. At the time of the first Earth Day, recycling was considered an eccentric activity of long-haired hippies and frugal New Englanders. Thirty years later, some municipalities fine you for *not* recycling, and schoolchildren are routinely taught the ecological facts of life. Thanks to federal legislation passed in the 1970s, DDT has been banned, lead has been removed from paint and gasoline, the air over many of our cities is cleaner, and rivers that once were clogged with industrial waste run more clearly. Many people have taken the message to heart and now use environmentally safe household cleaning products and energy-efficient light bulbs, drive hybrid cars, and support organic farmers.

There is still a lot to do. Even if you have cleaned up your home or your neighborhood, there are still larger issues to be addressed. Foremost among them is the exposure of our poorest children to the greatest number of toxins. Levels of lead, pesticides, solvents, mercury, particulates, and other forms of air pollution are all worst in low-income neighborhoods. We need to keep our eyes on the big picture and act both nationally and internationally. Pollution respects no boundaries, so by helping others, we help ourselves as well.

We consider environmental awareness to be a component of both integrative pediatrics and good parenting. Working for a cleaner environment affects not just our children's health today but also their health as adults, and the health of their children and grandchildren. We hope that all parents will try to protect their own children, and other children around the world as well, through whatever personal or political actions seem most suitable to their interests, time, and talents. Even the smallest steps help. For instance, the integrated pest-management program you help set up at your children's school to help reduce or eliminate the use of pesticides and herbicides may protect hundreds of kids now. The local campaign for lead abatement you devote some weekends to may allow generations of kids to reach their full intellectual potential. Little things can make a big difference and at the same time show our children the importance of conservation and protection of natural resources.

Physical Hazards

The environmental threats to your children's safety don't all come with polysyllabic chemical names. Some of them can be understood simply by imagining yourself an inexperienced, physically weak, low-to-the-ground being who is intensely curious about the world. Taking on that attitude as you stroll (or better yet, crawl) through the house will help you spot the unsafe things that can be opened, yanked on, pulled over, climbed up, fallen on, and otherwise interacted with by a youngster. If you maintain that attitude as you move around the yard or through the neighborhood, you'll see the greater risks they face because of their innocence, curiosity, or smaller size and strength.

Thirteen Ways to Keep Your Children Safe

1. *Buckle up*. Even a moderate-speed crash can turn unbuckled children into projectiles. If you insist on proper protection in the car, buckling up will eventually become an unconscious habit. Infants and children up to four years of age should always be in approved car seats in the back seat. Children up to 4' 9" tall or under 80 pounds need to use approved booster seats with their seat belts in the back seat—away from airbags. Young children using adult seat belts alone are four times more likely to suffer head, brain, and abdominal injuries in a crash than those using car seats or booster seats designed for them.

2. *Require bike helmets*. We've seen kids die in bike accidents, so as far as we're concerned, you're a neglectful parent if you allow your child to ride without a helmet. Helmets should be buckled securely and worn so they protect the forehead. You should wear your own, as well, while you're teaching your kids the basics of bike safety or enjoying a ride with them. Don't forget helmets for skiing, snowboarding, and sledding too.

3. *Avoid accidental poisonings*. Keep all toxic or caustic chemicals locked up, and that includes beauty aids like hair relaxers. Switch to nontoxic products when possible. Put supplements (even kiddie vitamins) and medications where children cannot ever reach them. Don't grow poisonous houseplants until the kids have stopped putting things in their mouths. Post the 800 number for poison control by the phone.

4. *Drownproof your kids*. Teach them how to stay afloat and then how to swim. If you have a pool, restrict access to it with a gate that locks. Put floatation devices on everyone on a boat. Always supervise young children in the bath—a child can drown in just a few inches of water. Carry a cordless phone with you to the pool or the bathtub, so you won't be tempted to leave a child alone in the water if the phone rings.

5. *Make sleep safe*. Lay your child on her back ("back to sleep") on a firm crib mattress—no soft mattresses, sofa beds, or water beds. Use only breathable blankets, rather than pillows or heavy quilts and blankets that can suffocate.

6. *Prevent fires*. Lock up matches. Keep fresh batteries in all smoke detectors, and install a carbon monoxide detector as well if you have a gas heater or appliances. Label your child's bedroom window with a decal that alerts firefighters to a child's potential presence. Practice fire drills as a family so everyone knows how to exit the house safely.

7. *Kidproof garage doors*. Either reduce pressure levels on old-style automatic doors so a child cannot be injured seriously if trapped beneath them, or install doors with electric eyes that halt the descent of the door when anyone breaks the beam of light.

8. *Do a safety survey of your home, looking at it from kid level*. Are there electrical or shade cords hanging, heavy potted plants or ornaments that can be tipped onto little heads, drawers or cupboards that do not lock? Are the handles of filled pots hanging out over the stove where kids can reach them? Is the hot-water heater set below 120 degrees to prevent burns?

9. *Look closely at toys*. Don't buy a child a toy that is not safe for her or his age. Watch out for foreign toys that may not meet U.S. safety standards.

10. *Use sunscreen on any child over six months of age to prevent burns now or skin cancers later in life*. Keep younger ones out of the sun except for short periods. Apply about a shot glass of SPF 15 to 24 sunscreen containing zinc oxide, titanium dioxide, or Parsol 1789 (avobenzone) to a child fifteen to thirty minutes before exposure, and every two hours thereafter. Reapply after swimming. Until more safety data become available, we recommend against using sunscreens and blocks containing nanoparticles.

Children should also wear hats, sunglasses, swim shirts, and other physical protection, especially during the hours of brightest sunshine from 10:00 AM to 4:00 PM. Remember that 80 percent of lifetime sun damage occurs before the age of eighteen—you don't want your kids to blame you for every wrinkle when they're middle-aged!

11. *Check playgrounds and playing fields for safety*. More than two hundred thousand preschool and elementary students go to the hospital Emergency Department every year for accidents sustained at playgrounds, and 36 percent of their injuries are serious ones. Avoid concrete and look for more forgiving surfaces like sand, bark, or the new rubberized asphalts. Make sure your children know how to use all the equipment safely, and that they are supervised at all times.

12. *Protect from abuse*. Be vigilant about who spends time with your child. Abuse by family, friends, and caretakers is a major cause of physical and emotional trauma for children.

13. *Wage peace*. Work with the neighbors and the police to create a safer neighborhood environment. Work with parents and teachers at your children's school to include the teaching of conflict-resolution and anger-management skills. And—it's a caution you only have to give in the United States—lock up firearms, unloaded, with the ammunition in a separate locked location.

CHAPTER 9

Aliens Are Brainwashing My Kids!

Protecting Your Children from Unhealthy Aspects of Popular Culture

Like fish through water, we move each day through a sea of cultural attitudes and directives. We are rarely even conscious of them, yet these cultural messages form our characters, influence our physical and mental health, motivate our actions, and contribute to our hopes and dreams. To adults much of this is just background noise—a sort of social static—but there is a far greater impact on our children, who have fewer defenses.

As physicians and fathers, we're deeply committed to protecting the minds, bodies, and spirits of vulnerable children. We believe some aspects of popular culture threaten the health of our youth psychologically and physically, and that it is important for doctors who care for children to speak out on this public health issue. For instance, the glorification of violence even in media aimed specifically at children has the end result of desensitizing many young people to the effects of violent behavior. The restaurant industry's suggestions that we supersize our meals contribute to both the obesity and the malnutrition of our children, with lifelong consequences. Dolls with unattainable dimensions and ubiquitous advertising that features waifish models make girls more susceptible to eating disorders. Similarly, unnaturally pumped-up action figures and buff male models put pressure on older boys to use steroids to achieve an idealized "manliness." Internet Web pages, blogs, and TV reality shows promote the concept that any behavior is OK as long as it gets you a little media exposure. And most of all, there is the stress of noise and overstimulation, of the pace of life, and of the pressure to be perfect.

Parents, doctors, and other advocates for children need to act together to protect our children from the cultural pressure to think or act in unhealthy ways. We counter this "mental pollution" best by instilling healthier messages about their selves, their families, their communities, and their world. It takes firmness and commitment, but we believe there are lots of ways that parents can insure they are the ones who have the major impact on their children's values and attitudes, not the mass media or the ubiquitous "everyone." We have the power to counterbalance the "Everyone says . . . ," "Everyone else has . . . ," and "Everyone else gets to . . ." messages our children are persistently exposed to.

There's no doubt that our kids are barraged with media images. The average child sees an estimated 360,000 television advertisements before graduating from high school—and that doesn't even count all the ads from the radio, the Internet, magazines, billboards, materials used in school, and even the logos plastered all over professional athletes. Children spend hours a day watching TV shows and logging onto Web sites that are often poor quality or not intended for their age group. How do kids make sense of all the information, misinformation, and manipulation they're exposed to through the media? It's your job to protect very young children from exposure to unhealthy messages and to teach older children how to analyze and understand the images beamed at them.

The first fact of life we have to accept is that the messages sent by the mass media are generally motivated by profit rather than a concern for what's best for our children. That's not evil—it's just the way it is. Our kids are a very desirable market, because all their income is disposable. Few parents realize the strength of this buying power, but American children under twelve spent nearly $18 billion dollars in 2006.

So we have a dangerous combination here—kids with lots of spending money who may not yet have developed the ability to discern fact from fiction. Many kids under the age of eight are developmentally unable to tell the ads from the TV shows, and they cannot grasp the concept that what they see in an advertisement may not be literally true. They don't have the tools to screen out the hyperbole and exaggeration that adults pretty much expect and ignore. Advertisers count on this developmental weakness and create materials to take advantage of it. In addition, kids see plenty of media messages supposedly aimed at adults. For instance, it's been estimated that 90 percent of the time children are watching TV they are looking at shows not intended for children.

The second fact of life is that images transmitted in the media have changed since we were children. There is certainly far more violence, sexuality, drug use, and bad language and attitudes in even PG-rated movies than there used to be, and TV shows and computer/video games have also ratcheted up the adult content in programs aimed at children and families. That's why it's so important to be familiar with the TV shows, songs, magazines, video games, and Internet sites to which your child is exposed. If you had assumed that the material on these media is what it was twenty or thirty years ago, when you were a kid, you'll be surprised by what you find. Even professional sports has changed, becoming more aggressive and more commercial and, in the case of professional wrestling, adding a sexual subtext where none existed before.

Countering Unhealthy Messages

As parents and community members we must make it a priority to model and instill in our children healthy values and behaviors. If we don't, they will assimilate the values and behaviors conveyed by the media and popular culture. They will grow up thinking that rich people are better, senior citizens are doddering fools, women are helpless, all family conflicts can be resolved in the ten minutes before the next commercial, and buying Nike shoes or drinking Gatorade will enable them to shoot and score like LeBron James.

We thought we would briefly tackle the cultural messages that we find most unhealthy and suggest ways parents can intercept or counter them. You may not agree with our choices—every family has its own values—but this short list is at least a way to start the conversation. It may also inspire a bit of soul searching of your own. All of us are affected by these toxic cultural influences too, and odds are our kids have picked up on them.

THE PROGRAMMING: *Money is everything. (Bling is the thing.)*

What's the number one value in America today? We'd have to say money, because that is so often the ultimate standard by which political, governmental, social, and commercial decisions are made. The bottom line determines whether we protect children from lead or not, whether we use fillers like sugar and salt in food or not, whether we add violence or sex to the movie or not, whether we pay day care workers and teachers well or not, whether we outlaw automatic weapons or not.

It is inevitable that children growing up in a society that worships the almighty dollar will receive this message in a thousand ways. As a result our kids seem to want to accumulate lots of the newest and most exciting "stuff." They scorn those who are not financially successful as "losers." They want to grow up to be rich and famous, preferably before the age of thirty and with the least possible expenditure of effort. But we don't want them to know the price of everything and the value of nothing, do we?

We are a nation that considers the word "consumer" synonymous with "person," where shopping is a major leisure-time activity. Popular culture tells us that we are what we buy, so many kids become overly concerned about having the "right" jeans and shoes and going to the "right" school. In a culture dedicated to consumption like ours, children are the ultimate marketing targets, in the hopes that the brand loyalty established in youth will continue for decades.

This cultural emphasis on the things that money can buy is especially harmful to those with limited financial resources. Struggling parents may find it painful or embarrassing that they cannot buy everything they would like to for the children they love, and that their children are teased or ignored by their peers for not having the right stuff. We think it's very important that parents who are financially comfortable teach their own children to offer kindness rather than derision to kids who cannot afford the latest fad.

Money doesn't automatically bring happiness, and it may not bring good health either. The latest research indicates that those who place great value on money and personal possessions are more anxious and depressed, have more physical complaints, and smoke and drink more than those who put more importance on their relationships with family, friends, and community.

▶ *The counterprogramming:* Help your children separate their "wants" from their "needs." Tell them you'll take care of their needs as you are able, but they may have to purchase things they want by saving their own allowances or earnings (or waiting till their birthdays). Find free activities to do as a family, like going to a park or a street fair. Encourage making rather than buying gifts. Share the beauty of simple things—a fresh blueberry, a starry sky, the smell of new-mown grass, an interesting detail on a building down the block. Strengthen their moral and spiritual values in whatever ways you can. A child with a strong spiritual center is less likely to worship money and material things.

Simplify your life. Gather together things you don't use (including toys) and donate them to a charitable organization. Involve your children in the service work you do and explain to them why you do it. Better yet, pick a special service activity for the entire family. Tell them stories about people who have performed admirable acts of charity. Don't audibly judge people by their possessions—or lack thereof. In a society that is increasingly breaking into "haves" and "have-nots," where one in six children live in relative poverty, it's important to teach your children compassion and understanding for those less fortunate than themselves. In our own homes, our children get excited about putting money into a jar for charity each week and deciding where to give the money when the jar's full.

Watch TV with your kids and comment now and then about what a product portrayed in an ad realistically can and cannot do to improve their lives. Teach your children how to be savvy shoppers so they don't confuse price for value, and show them that the most expensive item is not necessarily the best.

THE PROGRAMMING: *Speed is of the essence.*

Thanks to computers, e-mail, fax machines, and cell phones we are now living in an age when it is nearly impossible to be out of touch, and there is no longer any time to mull over an issue or an idea. We have become impatient with delay or with the slow pace of normal human interaction, and we often choose to do things quickly rather than thoughtfully. We become too focused on the destination and forget to enjoy the journey.

As we discussed in chapter 7, fast-paced living can be very stressful, especially if we don't make time to rest and rejuvenate. This applies not just to our day-to-day living but to our longer-term goals as well. Lots of parents are pushing their children to achieve more and faster in school, on the playing fields, in the arts—in nearly every area of their lives. They fill their children's lives with lessons and coaching and practice and tutoring. We say, "Give kids some time to be kids." They don't have to learn every possible skill and have every possible experience before they're eighteen. They need room to dabble, to try out new talents and experiences, to discover their own individual strengths and passions without the pressure to be the best or the most skilled. A tight focus too soon can actually stunt their creativity and resourcefulness.

A corollary to "speed is of the essence" is "you shouldn't have to wait for what you want." Granted, immediate gratification has its attractions, but a steady diet of getting whatever they want whenever they want it is a sure way to spoil kids. We're not talking about love and attention here, but about material things.

▶ *The counterprogramming:* See if you need to slow down the pace of life at your house. Let your children experience the emotional power of real, unhurried human interaction. Take the time to write them little notes or letters occasionally to express your delight or pride in something they've done. Read aloud, do puzzles, and play games together. Books on tape or CD, which require imagination and visualization to bring the story to life, might make a better, slower-paced babysitter than videos. Let your kids' interests and passions dictate how far or how fast they move in their endeavors.

Try not to indulge all of your children's material desires, as their wishes often change from day to day. Talk to your kids about your own long-term planning, about things you have struggled or worked for. Introduce school-age kids to the concepts of budgeting and saving. Require your children to put part of their earnings and allowance into short- or long-term savings and encourage them to save for a higher-priced item they really want.

THE PROGRAMMING: *The good life revolves around junk foods.*

The makers of unhealthy foods have a lot of power over our kids, who generally know very little about good nutrition. The advertising slots on children's programs are jammed with junk-food ads, creating a toxic health environment that encourages our kids not only to eat unwisely but to eat too often and too much as well. The restaurants themselves are everywhere. (You know you live in a rural area if the nearest

McDonald's or Wendy's is more than fifteen minutes away.) If that's not enough, they have playgrounds, special meals, and cheap toys to pull in the kiddies as well. Our kids are exhorted through the ads and reminded by the ubiquitous brightly colored buildings that food that is high in sugar, salt, fat, and calories and low in nutritional value is fun, tasty, and available all the time. As parents, we have to balance our children's longings for the unhealthy snack or quick trip to the drive-thru with our knowledge that such foods are linked to diabetes, cardiovascular disease, obesity, and cancer.

▶ *The counterprogramming:* Educate your children about nutrition in the ways we suggested in chapter 5. Help them deconstruct advertising appeals by the makers of junk foods. Find tasty, healthy snack foods that appeal to your children so they do not feel deprived by not having whatever new junk food is currently being heavily advertised. Steer them toward the healthier choices on the fast-food menus.

THE PROGRAMMING: *It's cool to be negative and disrespectful of others.*
The mass media is full of negative words and images. It depicts a world where the really cool kids are flip and uncaring and there's no percentage in being nice to anyone who can't do something for you. If you believe popular culture, only babies and other hopeless innocents have a positive attitude. (One need look no further than the widely popular *American Idol,* where Simon Cowell joyously separates performers from their self-esteem.) As a result, kids may think it's far more "adult" to be cynical and dismissive of traits like sincerity, kindness, courtesy, and joy and to look for a negative motivation behind every action. In fact, the primary method of communication for many older kids appears to be the put-down. As caregivers to children with special needs, we are especially horrified when we overhear someone described as "a retard."

Aside from the unpleasantness of dealing with a child who is always looking for the worst in a person or situation, negativity has real health effects. A cynical and disrespectful attitude fosters an unsupportive relationship with peers, family, and community that can undermine physical and emotional health. On the other hand, a positive attitude toward life is consistently associated with longer life, better health, and a more effective immune system.

▶ *The counterprogramming:* Teach your children to think more in terms of solutions rather than problems. If you take an optimistic approach to life yourself, your children are likely to imitate it. We're not suggesting you deny life's difficulties but merely that you pass on more of an "if life hands you lemons, make lemonade" attitude. That sort of thinking results in a more resilient person, one who is better able to survive and thrive despite the ups and downs of life. Encourage your children to treat people of all ages and backgrounds with respect and insist that others treat your kids with respect too. Praise acts of kindness. Don't make excuses for bad behavior, whether it's that of your own child or others. Point out celebrities or sports personalities who embody the values you wish to impart.

THE PROGRAMMING: *Looks are everything.*

This is not a new message, at least for females, who have for generations been under pressure to conform to (ever-changing) standards of beauty. However, this message is no longer aimed solely at adults but at adolescents of both sexes and younger kids as well. Now they too measure their worth by their appearance rather than attributes such as character or kindness. By giving them big-breasted, tiny-waisted Barbie dolls and G.I. Joes with giant pecs and biceps, we establish unattainable standards for body shape and set the stage for eating disorders and illegal steroid use during the teen years. The conflicting messages to stay slim and eat in unhealthy ways may well explain why so many American girls diet and why the percentage of girls who feel "happy with the way I am" drops from 60 percent in elementary school to 29 percent in high school.

▶ *The counterprogramming:* Expand definitions of beauty beyond those media darlings whose good looks have led them down dubious paths. Don't fall into the trap of allowing your child to be sexualized at too young of age. Point out to your kids not only physical characteristics like a man's attractive eyes, a woman's strong arms, or an elderly person's well-earned wrinkles, but also the less obvious beauties of a sharp mind, a sweet voice, or a courageous spirit. Be more concerned with your child's fitness and health than with whether he or she conforms to current standards of beauty. Make it clear you value strength of character over physical beauty.

THE PROGRAMMING: *Violent behavior is acceptable.*

Violent behavior is the norm in some places in America, and children suffer from it. Our inability to regulate guns puts too many children at risk at school and on the streets. Our inability to get a handle on child abuse means some are not even safe in their own homes. But even if they live in more peaceful surroundings, our children are still strongly influenced by the pervasive violence in the books, magazines, television, music, and movies that surround us. This physical, emotional, and verbal violence—often without consequence—can affect a child's understanding of "good" as opposed to "wrong" or even "evil," and it can cause unacceptable behavior when they copy aggressive moves in their play.

A heavy exposure to violent images can damage a child psychologically in three ways. It may make a child overly fearful of the world, it may make a child more aggressive, or it may desensitize a child to the pain and suffering of others. These images aren't just coming from certain kinds of music but from almost all forms of "entertainment," which are full of violent language and behavior. In our experience, teaching your children (especially boys) not to love violence is a very difficult thing, because that culture is so seductive. Through toys and video/computer games, powerless little kids get to blow up planets and yank the spinal columns out of "enemies." No one really gets hurt in this "play," but unfortunately the attitudes and actions practiced during these games can carry over into real life. "First-person shooter" video and computer games are worse than violent TV and movies because they require the player to identify with and assume the role of the aggressor, conditioning kids to seek violent solutions to conflict. (We don't worry as much about "slapstick violence" like that of the Three Stooges.)

Nurturing aggressive behavior has physical as well as psychological effects. Far from being a healthy outlet for aggression, violent video games raise levels of the same neurochemicals released by anger and hostility, emotions associated with lowered immunity and a wide range of cardiovascular problems. A recent study even found that hostile and aggressive young adults are more likely to already have changes in their arteries symptomatic of early atherosclerosis.

▶ *The counterprogramming:* Choose with your children the TV shows, videos, and computer/video games they will watch or play. Turn down the sound during commercials and talk about what you've seen. Pay attention to the lyrics of the songs your child listens to and discuss those that concern you. Let your children's friends' parents know not to show your child, for instance, a PG-13 or R-rated video without your permission.

If your child displays aggressive behavior, track down and deal with its inspiration. Teach your kids skills for resolving or avoiding conflicts. Let them know that anger is a natural emotion that can and should be controlled or channeled. Teach them to express it appropriately and to defuse it by counting to ten, going for a run, doing a breathing exercise, or writing in a journal. Show them lots of love and affection, and model the peaceful resolution of conflicts in your own relationships.

THE PROGRAMMING: *Cigarettes, alcohol, and certain drugs are glamorous.*

You may think the use of tobacco, drugs, and alcohol is not an issue for your child, but school counselors can tell you that these problems are occurring at younger and younger ages and across all social strata. It is not uncommon for middle-school students—even the ones from "good" families—to have to enter treatment for substance-abuse problems. Exposing the developing brain to these addictive substances may create a long-term need for the drug. The earlier you get hooked on tobacco or alcohol, for instance, the harder it is to quit. Don't think the tobacco and alcohol companies don't know this. Their ads may briefly warn about underage drinking or smoking, but they otherwise sure seem to be aimed right at young people.

▶ *The counterprogramming:* Evaluate your own use of alcohol, tobacco, and other drugs, and commit to being a good role model. Educate your kids, who may not understand the short- and long-term effects of substance use, or the permanence of some of these impulsive decisions. For instance, of the 5,000 kids who start smoking each day, 3,000 will become regular smokers and 1,000 will eventually die of a tobacco-related disease. Counter advertising that links smoking and drinking with popularity and desirability with the real effects of these drugs on their bodies—everything from bad breath, vomiting, and stupid behavior, to diseased organs and death.

Know your children's friends. Protect your children from peer pressure to try or use alcohol or tobacco by making sure their parties are always under parental supervision, and letting them know that it's OK to blame you for their not partaking. ("My dad would be furious if I did. And you know my dad. He'd find out.") Role-play situations with them so they have the tools to protect themselves when "friends" pressure them to use drugs or alcohol. Form alliances with other parents to provide safe drug- and alcohol-free places for kids to hang out, and let them know that you want to be told if they suspect your child has been smoking or drinking.

You cannot relax about substance abuse just because it was not an issue when you were a child. Alcohol, tobacco, and other drugs are now far more pervasive in the culture, are stronger, are less frowned upon, and are readily available—even in the schools.

THE PROGRAMMING: *Winning is everything.*

We love competitive sports, but as dads and coaches, we are often appalled by the messages adults send children about sports and sportsmanship. We have seen fathers (it's usually—but not always—the men) shout belittling comments to their own and other kids on the field, throw tantrums over how many minutes of game time or what position their kid will play, suggest ways to evade the rules, yell at the refs, and even threaten violence against players on the opposing team. A Florida youth sports league now requires all parents of potential players to take a one-hour class in appropriate conduct before their kid can even set foot on the playing field.

Adults need to back off and allow the children to enjoy themselves. Sports give kids the chance to experience the satisfaction of teamwork, the joy of camaraderie, and the thrill of achieving personal goals. The playing field is where they learn how to function in a group and to look out for and care for each other. The sense of sportsmanship and the enjoyment of physical activity they develop will stand them in good stead throughout their lives. It's a shame to spoil it all with a misguided desire to win at any cost. The reality is very few of our kids will go on to become highly paid professional athletes.

▶ *The counterprogramming:* Remember sports are play, and play is supposed to be fun. Make sure all kids get a chance to play and that players rotate positions so they all get a chance at the key ones. Watch your own behavior on the sidelines and feel free to criticize that of parents displaying the wrong attitudes. Praise good sportsmanship. Emphasize the specifics of play—a nice pass, a well-placed kick, good teamwork, the perfect double play—over the final score. Heap praise on children—on your team or the opposing team—who throw themselves fully into the game, regardless of whether they scored three times or not at all.

THE PROGRAMMING: *Sex sells.*

Our kids are being exposed to sexual messages at earlier and earlier ages. The "hooker look" of midriff-baring top and low-slung bottom is quite popular even in the under-ten crowd, and makeup kits for prepubescent beauty queens are everywhere. Children ape the sexual moves they see in music videos and movies without even knowing exactly what they mean. Even PG movies may contain sexual innuendo now. Our concern is that this early sexualization may encourage earlier sexual behavior.

▸ *The counterprogramming:* Help your children retain their innocence as long as you can by limiting the amount of trash they're exposed to. But don't leave them ignorant by delaying any talk about sex until they're teens. By then it may be too late. Encourage independence and resourcefulness in your daughters so they don't see sexual posturing as a way to get what they want or need. Buy them clothes that suit their age and the kind of behavior you want to encourage.

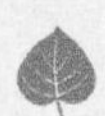

In this chapter we have tried to raise your awareness of what messages your children are picking up from the popular culture. Consider spending a little time looking at the world through your children's eyes. Read their magazines, watch the TV shows and videos they like, log on to their favorite Web sites, and listen to the songs on their playlists. You may decide to monitor their media input more than you did before (we recommend Internet filters) or change some of your own responses. Maybe as a result of reading this chapter you'll find the strength to not just throw up your hands in resignation and give in when your child keeps pressing for that 42-ounce Coke, the $100 name-brand jeans, or that R-rated teen-scream video. You may not always be the most popular parent in the house (or on the block), but parenting is not a popularity contest. Keep repeating the values you hold dear—and maybe, eventually, they will sink in.

[illegible]

In this chapter we have tried to raise your awareness of what messages your children are picking up from the [illegible]. Consider [illegible] a little time looking at the world through your children's eyes. Read their magazines, watch the TV shows and ads they like, go onto their favorite Web sites, and listen to the songs on their playlists. You may decide to monitor their media more than you did before (we recommend Internet filters) or change some of your own responses. Maybe [illegible] you'll find the strength to not just throw up your hands in [illegible] when your child [illegible]. [illegible] You may not always be the most [illegible] the parent [illegible]

SECTION II

therapies

CHAPTER 10

Little Bodies, Big Imaginations:

Mind/Body Medicine for Children

The term *mind/body medicine* may sound a little alternative, but both scientific research and clinical experience have repeatedly shown the effectiveness of therapies that activate the power of mind and spirit to help heal the body. These therapies work especially well in children and, in fact, were first embraced by pediatricians as safe, noninvasive ways to alleviate the pain or side effects of cancer therapy and chronic disease. Learning how to enlist emotions, attitudes, and thoughts in the healing process not only maximizes the good effects and minimizes the side effects of a conventional treatment, but it can also actually prevent or treat many conditions.

A certain amount of mind/body medicine is a part of every healing encounter—conventional or integrative. When your child's doctor tells her that a medication will make her feel better fast or sings a silly song to distract her from an incoming injection, that is mind/body medicine—whether the doctor is aware of it or not. When you watch a funny video to help you forget about what ails you, or when you take a few deep breaths before a stressful experience, you are practicing mind/body medicine. If you delivered your child using natural-childbirth methods, you have practiced mind/body medicine. Likewise when you kiss your little boy's "owie" to make it better, or hand your little girl her special "sleepy-time" teddy bear to help her fall asleep.

Doctors are now using mind/body techniques such as biofeedback and self-hypnosis to help children change unhealthy habits like bed-wetting, to ease pain, to relieve anxiety, to treat headache, stomachache, chemotherapy-induced nausea, and insomnia, to lessen the symptoms of asthma and irritable bowel syndrome, and even to cure warts.

Unlike Chinese, Indian, and many folk medicines, Western medicine has tended to treat the mind and the body as two completely separate entities. Integrative medicine acknowledges the connection between mind and body, with the causes of many medical problems falling on some point on the continuum between them. Some health conditions have a greater physical component, and some have a greater emotional and psychological component, but all have some of each. How can they not, when our brains, organs, and immune systems are in constant communication with each other?

The idea that what happens to the mind affects the body and vice versa is not so revolutionary. After all, many parents have seen stomachaches disappear as soon as the magic words "you can stay home from school today" are spoken—a fine example of physical pain caused by a stressful state of mind being cured when the source of anxiety or tension is resolved. You may also have had a toddler suddenly start wetting the bed again after a new baby is born. On the other hand, a physical problem can affect mental state. For example, an active child with an injury that precludes sports or play may become anxious or depressed when she cannot do all the things she is accustomed to doing.

Our entire medical system is based on the image of the body as a machine that can be fixed with the proper tool or intervention whenever it breaks down. Some scoff at the idea that their thoughts or emotions have anything to do with their physical health, but disease does not exist alone; it affects and is affected by a person's attitudes, lifestyle, thinking, and environment. When one part of the system falls out of balance, it naturally pulls on other aspects of the system, which must then also be addressed. You cannot deal successfully with the body without impacting the mind, and vice versa. Good doctors know this and frame their health advice carefully.

more on . . .

TESTING THE MIND/BODY THEORY

Want proof that what we think or feel can have a physical effect? Imagine holding a fresh, juicy lemon that you have just picked from the tree. Smell the lemon, drinking in its strong lemony aroma. Imagine that you are slowly cutting the lemon in half and that the juice is flowing down the sides of the fruit and onto your hand. Picture the bright yellow lemon half with drops of juice dripping from it. Now imagine biting into the sour, juicy flesh of the lemon. Your mouth is watering now, right? Just visualizing the lemon evoked a response from your salivary glands. In the same way, your heart beats faster and your senses go on alert when you read a Stephen King thriller late at night, even though there is no real danger threatening you. And haven't there been times in your life when repeating the familiar affirmation from *The Little Engine That Could* ("I think I can, I think I can") helped you do something you didn't think you had the strength to do?

Effective healers of all sorts know the power that belief—or lack of it—has in treatment. Doctors know that their patients respond better when they believe that their physician is skilled and caring. This is an example of the "placebo effect." A placebo (Latin for "I shall please") is a therapeutically inactive treatment, like the sugar pills once given to placate patients. Perhaps surprisingly, the placebo often causes an improvement or cure. For instance, parents often say to us, "You wouldn't know it to look at her, doc, but this child was sick as a dog just twenty minutes ago at home." Maybe it's the fresh air on the trip over, or the toys in the waiting room, but we think that the child's healing response has been activated by the sense that she is on the road to getting better. As fathers, we have learned the power of the words, "Don't worry, you'll start feeling better soon."

The placebo effect offers the purest example of a person's own innate healing capability, one that doctors usually take for granted. If you're wondering how a placebo can affect physical health when it is both harmless and inactive, you're not the only one. We think it's ironic that Western medical science dismisses the placebo effect as a nuisance that gets in the way of studying a drug instead of studying how to maximize the effectiveness of the placebo—which has no side effects at all. If we could harness or strengthen the placebo response, we would likely need to use fewer pharmaceutical drugs—or at least lower doses of them—and risk fewer side effects.

What Mind/Body Therapies Can and Cannot Do

Research into the mind/body continuum is really just coming of age in America, but we are slowly amassing data on the beneficial effects of such therapies as meditation/relaxation, biofeedback, hypnosis, guided imagery, and yoga. In addition to these clinical studies, researchers are looking more closely at the biochemical connections between the nervous, immune, gastrointestinal, and endocrine systems—body systems formerly thought to work independently of one another. It turns out that these four systems are actually in constant communication via hormones, brain chemicals, peptides, and other biochemical messengers. These signals go both from body parts to the mind and from the mind to the body, so that every physiological change in the body is accompanied by a change in mental and emotional state as well, and vice versa.

Using mind/body techniques, people can influence processes controlled by the autonomic (involuntary) nervous system that were once thought to be outside our control. For example, we can indeed alter such "unconscious" actions as blood pressure, breathing, heart rate, and circulation by learning to shift activity from the stimulating sympathetic arm of the autonomic nervous system to the more relaxed parasympathetic arm. We can influence other parts of the nervous system as well, changing our brain wave patterns or reducing or increasing our perception of pain. We can change the hormonal output from our endocrine systems and modify the balance between various immune cells. We can even improve intestinal function.

Mind/body medicine can sometimes be used to cure, especially those problems related to stress. It can also be used as a complement to conventional medicine to reduce pain, ease symptoms or drug side effects, and improve compliance with treatment plans. But it has its limitations, and some people go too far with the idea. While we strongly believe that the mind can influence the workings of the body and can certainly affect the immune system, we don't believe that the mind can cause disease—for instance, that we cause our own cancers by having pessimistic thoughts. Certain mind states such as stress may make a child more susceptible to disease, but his attitudes, beliefs, and emotions are not solely to blame when he gets sick. By the same token, if a child does not get better after using mind/body techniques, it does not mean that he has failed, or not tried hard enough. Every one of us is different, and what works for one may not work for another. The power of positive thinking cannot heal everything (though it will probably improve quality of life).

Mind/body medicine is often referred to in pediatrics as *self-regulation*. We like this term, as it suggests the power that a child holds in his own hands. It can be tremendously empowering for children to realize that they might be able to change the way they experience an illness or gain mastery over body processes they had thought to be beyond their control. In fact, just recognizing this possibility is enough to make some start to feel or function better.

Mind/body medicine should be a key component in any pediatrician's (and parent's) bag of tricks. We often see children with physical symptoms that upon examination have no medically explained physical cause, symptoms that we recognize as signals of psychological distress. For instance, stomach pain is a common complaint in children, who carry stress in their bellies, rather than in the head, neck, or back as adults do. Our patients are not faking or intentionally causing their tummy aches, but through mind/body techniques they can be taught how to consciously prevent or ameliorate them. Children are especially receptive to the idea that they have the power to help themselves and are generally better at the therapies than adults because they are more imaginative and open-minded. Their inexperience leaves them with no preconceived notions. There's no reason, to a child, why a special soothing pink seashell under the pillow won't bring sleep.

more on . . .

THE POWER OF THE PLACEBO

In studies, placebos have worked as well or better than the tested medications in trials of sedatives, antidepressants, and blood pressure drugs. In one placebo trial, people with asthma were told that one bottle of saltwater spray contained an allergen and another bottle of salt water contained a powerful allergy medicine. When exposed to the "allergen," 30 percent went into full-blown asthma attacks, and another 18 percent suffered airway restriction. Even more amazingly, in most cases their symptoms went away after they used the "drug." Smart health professionals try to use the power of the placebo to boost faith in any treatment.

We think it is helpful to introduce children to the concept of mind/body medicine when they are healthy so they have the proper mind-set in place and tools in hand when these techniques are needed medically. Any child can benefit from knowing mind/body approaches to reduce stress and anxiety when they arise. If you choose to use mind/body techniques for treatment, however, keep a few cautions in mind:

- *Rule out organic causes of illness*. Before you treat a child, say, for "school-day tummy," make sure it's not constipation, appendicitis, or inflammatory bowel disease.
- *Use mind/body techniques as a complement to*—and not a replacement for—drug or other medical therapies required by children with serious chronic diseases like asthma or juvenile rheumatoid arthritis.
- *Let the kid decide*. The choice to participate in any mind/body treatment must come from the children themselves, without parental pressure, because empowerment is an important aspect of healing.
- *Take care with more fragile kids*. The mind/body techniques of hypnosis and imagery should be used on children who have posttraumatic stress disorder, a history of abuse, or psychosis only by a specially trained therapist who knows how to handle any unsettling emotions or images that may come up.

A certain percentage of children tend to experience psychological distress as physical symptoms. Children who frequently experience headache, fatigue, dizziness, stomachaches, or chest pain for which no organic cause is found may be "somatizers" who are actually suffering from anxiety, depression, or antisocial disorders. The source of their distress needs to be uncovered through other means, such as counseling, after which the child can be taught mind/body strategies to help her cope.

Use of mind/body therapies has become quite commonplace in pediatrics in the past twenty years, perhaps more so than in any other field of medicine. We actually use mind/body medicine in some form or another in every encounter with a patient, even if it is only in the way we phrase questions or advice to elicit the greatest healing response.

- We evoke the positive powers of the placebo by the attention we pay, the efforts we take to increase our patients' control over their conditions, and our confidence in the efficacy of the treatment we have advised.

- We ask our small patients what *they* think the cause of their problem is—and what they think might help—in order to discover and utilize their hopes and fears in our therapy. These insights can, for example, help a patient with chronic problems alter the experience of the illness and thereby alleviate some of its symptoms.

- We use specific techniques, such as breath work, self-hypnosis, music, or distraction to lower anxiety or perceived pain during office procedures like blood draws or shots.

- We also use or refer patients to other practitioners for various mind/body therapies to treat specific conditions, as we will discuss in Section III.

We believe that techniques such as breathwork, relaxation, meditation, hypnosis, guided imagery, yoga, counseling, and the creative arts can offer great benefits to our patients. We aren't expert in all the techniques we'll be discussing in this section. We do practice most of them and are well enough versed in the others to be able to devise an integrated treatment plan and refer our patients to skilled practitioners. We can tell you what each technique is and how it is used. Where we can, we'll give you a sample activity so you can get a taste of the therapy. Some of these techniques require training, some require the presence of a therapist or technician, but most can be done by you and/or your child whenever and wherever suits you. Using these tools will let your child—the one who always says, "I want to do it for myself"—assume greater control of his own body.

The most important factor in successfully using a mind/body therapy with children is the wholehearted support of both children and parents. Some parents are not comfortable with some forms of mind/body medicine due to their religious or world views. We try to be sensitive to signs of parental apprehension or disbelief, so we can discuss these concerns openly with the parents and answer all questions. We want to make sure that the parents understand the cause of their child's health problem and are supportive of our proposed treatment. For the same reasons, parents and children need to feel confidence and trust in the person conducting the mind/body sessions. If there is not good rapport between child and practitioner, the child may not be able to relax deeply enough to focus on the training.

The Mind/Body Toolbox

For ease of discussion, we have divided mind/body therapies into three categories of tools:

- *Pocket tools* that are always with your child and can be used any time
- *Tools that are kept in the drawer* because they require some parental supervision or assistance, at least in getting started
- *Power tools*, or techniques that should be learned under the direction of a trained practitioner

In our experience, many parents need these tools as much as their children do, so consider practicing some of these mind/body techniques as a family.

Pocket Tools

In this category we include methods of stress reduction that children can access and use on their own at any time, such as breath work, muscle relaxation, social and family support, journaling, and exercise. In addition to these specific therapies, it is helpful if parents and other mentors can teach children attitudes and skills that increase their ability to solve problems and give them a sense of mastery. A feeling of mastery is important in developing the optimistic attitude associated with longer life and better physical and mental health. Caring adults can teach children how to be their own coaches, engaging in positive self-talk ("I can do it!") that encourages an upbeat, healthy attitude. In fact, one of the most powerful pocket tools may just be laughter.

Breath Work

Even though breathing is essential to life, few of us pay any attention to doing it right. We breathe shallowly and high in our chest, which doesn't provide much oxygen for our body's cells and tissues or keep breathing muscles like the diaphragm toned. Some of us forget to breathe at all, especially when we are concentrating.

Yet it turns out that the simple act of breathing in and out can have powerful effects on the body. For this revelation, we should thank the yogis of India, who pioneered the study and practice of breath work, learning to control body functions such as hunger, thirst, blood pressure, heart rate, and temperature as part of their spiritual practice. In India the word for "breath," *prana*, is also the word for "spirit." In English, the words "spirit" and "respiration" share the same Latin root.

The breath, being a part of both the voluntary and involuntary nervous systems, is able to affect both the body and the emotions. Proper breathing can calm the nervous system, slow the heart rate, stimulate the immune system, and even switch your mind over to another form of brain wave. As the esteemed yoga teacher B. K. S. Iyengar once said, "Regulate the breathing and control the mind." Imagine—you can control how you feel physically, emotionally, and mentally with your breath! That's a lot of power. Breathing in certain ways can make you feel more positive, more alert, and more energetic, or it can make you feel calmer and more relaxed. The trick is to pay attention, to be aware of your breath, of how you breathe, and how fast. When you breathe in and out slowly and deeply, you relax and release anger and muscular tension. When you breathe quickly and powerfully for a few seconds, you may feel more alert.

Breath work can be used to relieve stress, pain, panic, or anxiety and can make you more aware of what's going on in your own body. When we give a shot or draw blood, we distract our patients from fear or pain by asking them to pay attention to their breath or blow soap bubbles. We teach slow deep breathing to kids with asthma to help them prevent, or reduce the severity of, asthmatic attacks. We use what is called diaphragmatic breathing, or belly breathing, to help children slow their heart rate, reduce pain perception, and calm their nervous system. It's simple and easy to learn (see the box below), as long as you remember to let your stomach relax and pooch out a little rather than holding it in. We also described several breathing exercises in the box on mini-relaxation exercises in chapter 7.

Intentional Muscular Relaxation

Many children—and their parents—unconsciously spend their days with their muscles clenched. This muscle tension inhibits circulation and allows toxic waste products to build up in the tissues, causing pain and slowing healing. Intentional muscular relaxation techniques help you discover where tension is being held in your body and allow you to release it. The techniques themselves simply call for tightening and then relaxing the muscles in the body. Many people find that these exercises offer them a chance to finally feel what it's like to be totally relaxed.

BELLY BREATHING

Have your child put her hand gently over her belly button. Ask her to imagine that she has a balloon underneath her belly button that will blow up when she inhales. Ask her to breathe in through her nose slowly to the count of three or four, pulling the air deep into her lungs and feeling her belly expand like a balloon blowing up. Make sure her shoulders are loose and relaxed. Now ask her to breathe out through her mouth slowly to a count of six or eight, feeling her belly deflate like a balloon. Tell her to take her time. Young children can do this for a minute or two, gradually working up to ten to twenty minutes, as they get older.

Adapted from Rebecca Kajander, *Diaphragmatic Breathing* (1997)

LETTING GO OF TENSION

Floppy Raggedy Ann or Andy: This is a good exercise for helping a child become aware of just how a relaxed body feels. Ask your child to imagine herself a floppy rag doll. Everything should feel loose and comfortable. Tell her to let herself be all floppy like Raggedy Ann. Pick up an arm and praise her for the way it flops down when you pick it up. Now check the other arm, and praise its floppiness. Encourage her to be loose and floppy like Raggedy Ann all over.

Progressive muscular relaxation: We recommend playing this as a kind of Simon Says game with your child. First, ask the child to lie down in a comfortable position. Ask him how the muscles in his body feel. Are they loose? Tight? Ask him to clench each part of his body for five to seven seconds and then release, breathing throughout the exercise, and then taking a nice big breath before he moves on to the next body part. Start with the toes, then gradually do the feet, ankles, calves, stomach, fanny, chest, fingers, hands, arms, shoulders, throat, and all parts of the face. Then have him tighten everything at once for seven seconds and release. Ask him how his muscles feel now.

Adapted from Karen Olness and Daniel Kohen, *Hypnosis and Hypnotherapy with Children* (1996), and Herbert Benson, *The Relaxation Response* (1976)

Exercise

We devoted an entire chapter (chapter 6) to the healthy effects of exercise, but we would like to remind you again that physical activity can affect the mind and the emotions. Exercise is a proven stress reducer and mood elevator. When your child is stressed, depressed, or angry, suggest a quick walk to blow off steam, a game of Frisbee, dancing to favorite music, or even ten minutes of just charging up and down the stairs.

Journaling

Keeping a diary or a journal can help reduce stress and ease physical and emotional pain by giving a child a safe place to disclose or explore worrisome thoughts. Your child might want to have his own journal (don't peek), or you might keep a family or parent/child journal that allows family members to express themselves emotionally on paper when it is hard to do so face-to-face. Younger children may enjoy journaling in the form of a poster that keeps track of progress (dry nights, servings of fruits and vegetables eaten) toward certain goals with stars or other fun stickers or stamps. Positive reinforcement like this can be very helpful in changing behavior.

Social Connections

Study after study has found that people who are loved by their families, supported by their friends, and involved in their communities live longer and healthier lives. Positive social interactions with others not only bring value and meaning to our lives, but they relieve stress, build support systems, and prevent isolation. Some people with chronic health problems even find that they feel less pain while having fun with friends or doing volunteer work. There are a million ways to build healthy connections within your family through family rituals, meetings, meals, and trips. Children can also build their own social and emotional support systems through team sports, extracurricular activities, volunteer activities, and correspondence with age-appropriate online pals or distant friends and family.

Tools in the Drawer

Tools in the drawer require a little guidance or training. You and/or your children might need to take a class to get started or turn to the resources section at the end of the book for lists of organizations, books, tapes, or Web sites that may be helpful to beginners. We heartily recommend both yoga and meditation as activities that are even better when done as a family.

Yoga

Here in the West, few of us use the full range of yoga practices promoted in the East. We focus mostly on the use of meditative awareness, breathing exercises, and physical exercises (called postures, or *asanas*) to help reduce stress and improve fitness, flexibility, and mood. Although the health benefits of yoga have been long studied in Asia, we have only just begun to do research on the subject here. So far in the West, yoga has been shown to be useful for conditions like asthma, sleep disorders, and some cases of chronic pain such as migraine headaches.

Yoga can be fun with kids of any age. Very young children can do yoga for short periods. As they grow older they can hold the poses longer and with greater precision. You might find, to your chagrin, that your own little lions and cobras are far more flexible than you are.

YOGA ANIMALS

Kids love the dramatic possibilities of the postures named after animals and the fun of imitating Mom or Dad. After some gentle warm-up activity, repeat each exercise three times (sound effects optional). For illustrations of poses, use one of the books listed in Resources.

The Cobra: Lie face down on the floor and relax. Place your palms on the floor next to your upper chest, elbows close to your sides. Slowly raise your head and neck, gently pushing up with the hands so your back curves up while your belly button or hip bones remain on the floor. Look up without straining your neck. Make a hissing noise like a snake and maybe some snaky tongue movements. Hold the pose for five to ten seconds, breathing easily, and then slowly return to the floor.

The Cat: Get down on your hands and knees with your hands right under your shoulders and your knees right under your hips. Take a deep breath. As you breathe in, slowly arch your back like a cat, curling your head down and tucking in your tailbone. Purr if you like. As you breathe out, slowly raise your head and lift your tailbone, so your spine curves in an easy backbend and your tummy reaches for the ground. Give a few meows. Go gently back and forth between the two poses a few times, slowly and smoothly.

The Lion: Sit on your folded legs with your butt resting on the back of your heels. Rest your hands on your knees. Take a deep breath and, keeping your head straight, open your mouth wide and stick your tongue out as far as you can. Give a mighty ROAR! Take another deep breath and roar, repeating three times.

Meditation

You don't need to find a guru or go to a monastery to meditate. In fact, although forms of meditation are an important part of several religious traditions, when doctors and researchers talk about meditation, they have something more secular in mind. They are referring to the self-directed process of focusing on a sound, an image, or a thought to still the mind and relax the body. Dr. Herbert Benson of Harvard University's Mind/Body Institute called his meditative technique "the relaxation response" specifically to rid this stress-reduction tool of any religious implications. You can choose to meditate in a way that delivers a spiritual benefit as well (Benson himself thinks that deepens its effect), but that's up to you.

Studies of meditation in adults have found that regular meditation can lower blood pressure, improve heart health, relieve pain, and reduce anxiety. As integrative doctors, we have recommended meditation for reduction of both pain and stress, as well as for complementary therapy for autoimmune and breathing disorders. There is little clinical evidence on the effects of meditation on children, but in our experience (and that of other practitioners) children can also benefit from regular meditative practice, which then becomes a tool they can take into their adult lives to help stay centered and balanced.

BASIC MEDITATION

Sit in a quiet place in a comfortable position. Close your eyes, and relax your muscles. Breathe slowly and repeat your focus word or phrase silently in your mind. If your attention wanders, draw it back to your focus word. Don't be worried or irritated, just gently return to saying your word in your mind. Do this for five minutes at first, then extend the time as you are able. When the time is up, open your eyes. Sit for a minute or two to enjoy the feeling of relaxation before going on about your day.

Adapted from Herbert Benson in *Mind Body Medicine* (1992)

HINT: A child's ability to meditate increases with age. A preschooler may only be able to handle a few minutes at a time, whereas a middle-school child could meditate for ten to fifteen minutes once or twice a day. Consistency of practice is important. The more you meditate, the better you get at it.

There are many ways to meditate, and no single way is the "right" way. You have to discover what's right for you and your child. Many people meditate in a comfortable seated position, but some meditate while walking. Some meditators focus on a meaningful word or phrase ("peace," or "love," for instance), others on an image, like a starry sky or a loved one's face. Those practicing what is called *mindfulness meditation* don't focus at all, allowing thoughts to drift across the mind without getting involved in them. Meditation can be done alone or in groups, at a regular time of day or whenever it's needed, seated or walking, in long stints or short bursts, with music or in silence.

Power Tools

Power tools call for the help of a trained practitioner. Once a child is trained, however, he or she will be able to use the skills at will. Although there are other useful techniques that also fall into this category—such as art, dance, and music therapy—they are not often used in primary care and so we are less familiar with them. We will be focusing instead on biofeedback and the various forms of self-hypnosis and visualization—power tools that we use extensively in caring for our patients.

TIP: One way to introduce focused quiet time to young children is to play a dreamy instrumental CD and ask your kids to close their eyes and breathe in and out gently. Ask them to picture the sky, a river, or a favorite animal while the music plays for three to five minutes. Then they can open their eyes, feeling relaxed and refreshed.

Biofeedback

This is a heavily used therapy in pediatrics, and there's a lot of clinical evidence of its effectiveness. The power of biofeedback comes not just from teaching kids how to make actual physiological changes in their bodies but also from the graphic proof it gives children that they can have mastery over their physical conditions—that they are not the powerless victims of their bodies.

Biofeedback uses sensitive machines to monitor body processes and display the information via sounds or pictures. Biofeedback machines can be set up to respond to increases or decreases in heart rate, muscle tension, peripheral body temperature, sweat-gland response, or brain wave activity. The machine makes visible what is normally invisible, so that a child can see what is happening in her body and learn how to influence it. The various systems of our bodies communicate with each other all the time. Biofeedback allows us to open these messages and—with an increased awareness of body sensations—change what they say. Once a child learns how these self-regulatory skills feel and has practiced them both with and without the machine, the machine is no longer necessary except as an occasional refresher.

In a first session a health professional trained in biofeedback will talk with your child about the goals of treatment—for instance, to reduce the severity of asthma attacks. He will explain what body function the child will be trying to affect, and he will apply sensors hooked to the computer to various parts of the body depending on what physiological factor will be measured (muscle tension, respiration, etc.). The computer may communicate this information through a readout, a sound, or a computer game. The child then attempts to change the body function in the desired way, using the computer feedback.

Children learn especially quickly with biofeedback, which is often described as "a video game for your body." In fact, the computerized games used in many biofeedback programs for children make sessions fun and involving. For instance, kids can learn how to tense and relax specific muscle groups to determine the path of a computer spaceship trying to avoid asteroids. Children may become competent in self-regulation after a month of once-a-week, 40- to 60-minute biofeedback sessions (younger children will have shorter sessions), and maintain their skills through home practice and the occasional follow-up.

Biofeedback is recommended for a variety of pediatric conditions, often in combination with self-hypnosis or relaxation. The self-regulation skills learned by children through biofeedback have been found to help reduce the number, severity, and duration of migraine and tension headaches; improve circulation in their hands and feet to counter the effects of Raynaud's syndrome; ease problems of muscular tension; relieve the pain of cancer, burns, or arthritis; and manage anxiety. We'll discuss some of these uses in Section III.

Self-Hypnosis, Visualization, and Guided Imagery

We discuss these three therapies together because there is so much overlap in their use and effect. They all evoke a trance state of higher alertness that focuses concentration and allows access to the unconscious mind. While training and credentials vary in this field, all three therapies take advantage of the fact that images created in the mind can seem as real to the body as those actually experienced. By allowing mind and body to "talk" to each other through words and images, these therapies offer children a child-controlled, child-centered way of managing habits, regulating some aspects of body function, and activating their own healing powers.

Hypnosis may rely more on the words of the therapist for its effects, and visualization/imagery may depend more on the patient's own images and perceptions, but in truth there are more similarities than differences in these techniques. In fact, a practitioner of clinical hypnosis may use imagery both to invoke a trance state and to offer suggestions during it. We advise parents to look for a physician, psychologist, or other health professional trained in clinical hypnosis or guided imagery. If there is no one with appropriate training in your area or cost is an issue, you may have to resort to a good book or audiotape/CD specific to your child's problem and work with her yourself, hopefully with her doctor's guidance.

A practitioner trained in clinical hypnosis will not make your child stand up and bark like a seal or implant a post-hypnotic suggestion that will make her do something stupid or embarrassing later. That's show biz, not medicine. The kind of therapeutic hypnosis we're talking about is just a tool that allows communication with emotions and thoughts buried in the unconscious that may be affecting your child's health or behavior. Children are always in control during their sessions, and they come out of or change the content of imagery or hypnotherapy sessions whenever they want, just as they can change their daydreams.

more on . . .
THE TRANCE STATE

A trance is not as exotic as it sounds. Kids move in and out of trance states all day. When they sit open-mouthed in front of the TV or computer screen, they're in a trance state. When they are so engaged in a book or a piece of music that they don't hear you call them for dinner, they're in a trance state. Hypnosis and imagery merely take advantage of this state of relaxed body/alert mind to use your child's imagination and concentrated attention to intentionally heal or to change behavior.

Children have so few filters and such active imaginations that they can usually get into a receptive state very easily and safely. In fact, there's already a component of hypnosis in your child's encounters with the doctor. We're not talking about Jedi mind tricks here, but the fact that children are usually very focused on the doctor from the minute they walk into our examining room. Whether it's from fear, curiosity, or respect, that intense focus makes them very susceptible to our suggestions. As young doctors we used to be puzzled by parents' reports that our offhand advice to their children about simple problems like wetting the bed or sleeping in their own beds invariably led to improvement. With experience and professional growth, we have come to see that we were overlooking a powerful tool.

Many doctors and other medical/dental professionals have learned to use simple imagery exercises to relax children or relieve the pain of a procedure. In addition, they may refer patients in need of more intense or focused therapy to people trained in clinical hypnosis or guided imagery. Professionals skilled in hypnosis or imagery can give a child the tools to relieve pain, reduce anxiety, heal faster after surgery, reduce the side effects of chemotherapy, stop bad habits like bed-wetting and nail-biting, sleep better, ease asthmatic breathing, and make rashes and other skin problems disappear.

The purpose of hypnosis or visualization is to strengthen *self-control*. The specialist is merely the coach who teaches the child how to regulate her behavior and body processes. During a session, this "coach" will first spend a little time developing rapport with your child and discussing the problem to be addressed. Then your child will be guided into a relaxed trance state in order to access those emotions and thoughts that cannot be reached through the conscious. This state may be accessed through simple diaphragmatic breathing and/or an imagery exercise that mentally takes the child to a favorite place or activity. In hypnosis, questions will be asked, and suggestions to help the child achieve goals of self-regulation may be offered.

These will be suggestions, not directives; your child remains in control. Someone who specializes in visualization or guided imagery will rely on sensory information—images, taste, smell, sound, and touch—rather than words, in the belief that the brain communicates more easily through images. The images will be explored for their meaning. Using words or images, the child can learn how to be more aware of what's happening in her body and then be coached into visualizing step-by-step the successful achievement of a behavioral goal (staying dry all night) or the physical changes she wants to occur (bronchial tubes as wide-open superhighways). She can also be taught how to imagine herself in a safe favorite place whenever she needs to separate herself from pain. After training, your child can do her visualization exercises or self-hypnosis alone, with your help, or with a CD or audiotape. In studies, even children as young as three have been able to learn these techniques, although skill increases with age.

FINDING YOUR SAFE PLACE

A visualization session may start with a relaxing exercise like this one:

▶ Allow yourself to imagine a comfortable place, a peaceful place. It might be a place you've been before or somewhere that's just coming into your imagination now. Just pick the first place that comes to mind.

▶ Allow yourself to imagine that you are in that place right now. If you want, describe what you imagine. What do you see? How do you feel? What is the temperature? What time of day is it? What do you hear or smell? How does the ground feel under your feet?

▶ Find a spot in that place where you feel most comfortable. Spend a few minutes enjoying the sensations you experience there. (The session continues from this point.)

Counseling

We are big fans of counseling, and we refer patients and/or their families to it with some regularity when issues arise where an objective, well-trained, and experienced outside voice can be invaluable, for both child and parent. School or private therapists can help a child give voice to fears, perceptions, or sadness in a comforting environment and can help open lines of communication that ease misunderstanding, anguish, and other ailments both physical and spiritual.

Families are sometimes resistant to the suggestion of counseling, as they view anybody who goes through therapy to be "crazy." We often point out that the only dysfunctional families we deal with are those that refuse help in the form of counseling when it is needed. There are many forms of counseling, including music and art therapy and short-term cognitive-behavioral therapy (CBT), so you should be able to find a style and a practitioner to suit your situation. Look for a therapist who comes with recommendations and an upstanding reputation. We recommend sitting in during the first few sessions to assess the approach of the therapist and encourage an environment of trust and safety.

How to Give Your Child a Magic Feather

In the classic Disney cartoon *Dumbo*, the big-eared baby elephant cannot fly until he is given a "magic" feather. He always has the ability to fly, but he has been grounded by his lack of belief in himself. There may be times when your child needs a "magic feather." He may have school-morning tummy or sleeping problems or difficulties sticking with a prescribed regimen for asthma. She may be nervous about the big game or a move to a new home. A little mind/body medicine may help.

Here are a few tips for helping your child activate mind/body responses:

- Make it clear that you have faith in your child and his ability to prevail over adversity. Your support is the most powerful magic feather a child can have.

- Be vocal in your support for the healing program your pediatrician has proposed. Encouraging your child's belief that she will be cured optimizes the healing response by calling upon the power of the placebo.

▶ Encourage a sense of health. Congratulate your child on having a strong and healthy body. Point out how quickly his cuts heal.

▶ Ask about feelings and emotions when children are ill or anxious. Help them understand that sometimes our emotions are expressed through our bodies. What's going on at home or school? Talking to a teacher or school counselor may be helpful.

▶ Establish healing rituals. Use prayers, symbols, mantras, or imagery sessions to support your child's wellness.

▶ Take a positive approach to healing, using affirmative statements rather than negative ones. The unconscious mind does not recognize negative words like "no" and "not" and so is likely to hear, "I will not pee in my bed in the middle of the night," as "I will pee in my bed in the middle of the night." It is far better to frame the statement as, "I will stay dry all night."

CHAPTER 11

The Healing Touch:

Manual Medicine

In the last chapter, we talked about mind/body medicine, or how abstract things like thoughts and feelings can affect your children's physical health in concrete ways. In this chapter we talk about therapies that rely on the physical—touch, movement, or manipulation—to improve mood, build immunity, treat disease, and create a sense of overall balance and wellness.

So what is manual medicine? We use the term to encompass both osteopathy—a complete system of medicine for primary care—and such stand-alone techniques as chiropractic, massage, exercise, and various forms of bodywork. These modalities use physical movement and/or touch to:

- *Relieve muscle tension*. This can reduce pain, improve circulation, boost immune function, and change unhealthy patterns of movement or behavior.

- *Express caring, or transmit healing energy*. Many doctors today have become so dependent on science that they have forgotten the healing power of a hand held or a shoulder patted in a reassuring manner.

- *Restore systemic balance*. Most practitioners of manual medicine have an integrative point of view and believe that injury or imbalance in one organ or body system causes or is reflected in imbalances in other systems as well.

- *Restore energy flow that has been blocked by physical or psychological trauma.* Cranial osteopathy and manual techniques from Chinese medicine such as acupressure and *tui na* are most commonly used for this purpose.

- *Heighten awareness of body function and increase alertness to important body cues.*

- *Encourage appreciation of the pleasure of nonsexual touch.* Therapies like massage teach children to feel comfortable with touch and to understand its healing power. If they learn to give massage as well, they have another way to exercise compassion.

- *Create a healthy sense of body image and acceptance of oneself.*

- *Access the unconscious.* Some forms of bodywork are based on the theory that memories (often painful) are stored not only in the mind but also as patterns in muscle, collagen, organs, and other tissues. Manipulation of the body releases these stored experiences, allowing unhealthy physical, mental, and emotional behavior to be changed.

In this chapter we will introduce you to the forms of manual medicine we think most useful to help prevent or treat disease in children. In our experience, children respond especially well to these therapies, because they haven't yet formed any adult biases against them. We'll start with osteopathy, which is a complete system of medicine, and then deal with those body/mind tools that can be used as a complement to conventional medicine.

Osteopathic Medicine

Many people do not know what an osteopathic physician is, and might even be surprised at the inclusion of the word "physician" in the title. But, in fact, we have two kinds of "approved" conventional medicine in this country—allopathic medicine and osteopathic medicine—with similar training and accreditation. Osteopathic physicians, or D.O.s (doctors of osteopathy), go through college, four years of medical school, internship, and usually years of specialist training just as M.D.s (medical doctors) do. They are licensed to prescribe drugs and to perform surgery, and have hospital privileges. Most provide primary care as family practitioners, internists, pediatricians, or gynecologists, but many specialize in areas such as surgery or anesthesiology. In short, they have similar training and licensure and can provide the same breadth of care as M.D.s. Once labeled a "cult" by the American Medical Association, these early advocates of integrative medicine are now well regarded, and their numbers are growing, especially in underserved rural areas.

Osteopathic training traditionally has one essential component that conventional medicine lacks—a belief that the structure and function of the body are intimately related, and that careful application of the hands in a therapeutic manner can restore balance and enhance healing. In addition to the usual curriculum, osteopathic physicians are also taught how to prevent, diagnose, and treat illness with their hands, using a series of techniques called *osteopathic manipulative treatment* (OMT). Their use of touch allows them to be more alert to asymmetry, restrictions in range of motion, and abnormalities of texture that might indicate dysfunction, and to treat them by manipulating muscles, joints, and other tissues to restore normal function.

As you can imagine, we find a lot to like in the osteopathic philosophy, and we are just as comfortable recommending an osteopathic physician as a medical doctor for the primary care of your children. Our preference is for practitioners who still follow the traditional philosophy and methods of osteopathic manipulation. Unfortunately, such practitioners are a bit of an endangered species. Only a small percentage of D.O.s still use OMT in addition to conventional care. Even fewer perform cranial osteopathy, the diagnostic and manipulative technique we find most interesting from a pediatric point of view.

We have been impressed by the healing potential for CO that we have seen in our own practices. We sometimes refer patients for cranial osteopathy for recurrent ear infections, headaches, sinus or respiratory problems (including asthma), learning disabilities, and attention deficit disorder.

more on . . .

CRANIAL OSTEOPATHY

The concepts underlying cranial osteopathy (CO) are quite controversial, with little data yet to support them, but the approach is extremely gentle, and we have witnessed some remarkably positive effects on some children. Osteopaths believe that cerebrospinal fluid normally moves up and down within the spinal column between the sacrum ("tail-bone") and the brain with a subtle pulse called the cranial rhythmic impulse (CRI) that is similar to and as important as the more obvious rhythms of blood flow and breath. This pulse, they say, is reflected in barely perceptible movement of the bones of the head and face, sacrum, and associated body membranes. Minor falls and accidents or trauma incurred during birth may restrict this natural expansion and contraction, causing an imbalance in the body that can lead to a range of pediatric and adult conditions from colic to learning and behavioral problems.

A treatment with CO starts with a gentle, hands-on examination to evaluate the cranial rhythmic impulse and pinpoint any restrictions in the movement of cerebrospinal fluid. Then extremely light pressure is used to release any restrictions in the sacrum, head, or facial bones, restoring movement to the bones and balance to the body as a whole.

If you decide to try this therapy for your child, look first for an osteopathic physician, because CO is typically an integral part of their philosophy and training. If you cannot find an osteopathic physician skilled in cranial osteopathy near you, look for an M.D., dentist, or other allied health professional with pediatric experience trained at a reputable school in cranial osteopathy or in a related stand-alone technique called craniosacral therapy (CST).

Chiropractic

Back pain is such a common symptom in this country that most adults are familiar with the kind of care offered by a chiropractor. We're used to lying on the special table while the chiropractor works on our spines, and many of us have experienced great relief from these treatments. But how useful is chiropractic care for children, for whom back pain is a less common problem?

Chiropractors are now the third-largest group of practitioners in the country (after medical doctors and dentists). Doctors of chiropractic (D.C.) are licensed in all fifty states after four years of medical training with a focus on spinal manipulation. Chiropractic medicine is based upon the belief that most illness arises from misalignments of the spine (subluxations) that impede the free flow of life energy through the nervous system. By using physical manipulation to return the vertebrae to their proper place, chiropractors try to rebalance this life energy and restore optimal function to the nervous system, which in turn promotes proper function in all organs and systems.

A small percentage of chiropractors ("straights") still believe that spinal adjustments cure all disease. Another small group ("evidence based") restricts itself solely to those musculoskeletal complaints for which spinal adjustment has been scientifically proven to be effective. Most chiropractors nowadays, however, are "mixers" who acknowledge other causes of disease and may use botanicals, nutritional supplements, physical therapy, homeopathy, and/or other techniques in addition to spinal adjustment.

In adults, chiropractic is now considered an effective therapy for the treatment of acute low back pain, and many people report it to be of use for neck pain as well. However, there is very little research on the use of chiropractic on children. Although chiropractors are now treating children for asthma, allergies, ear infections, colic, bed-wetting, and other disorders, there are few studies yet to prove benefit (and some studies showing no benefit at all).

The chiropractic profession is currently engaged in outreach to establish themselves as "gatekeepers to the health care system" and increase the number of children under their care. While we respect the field and acknowledge that there are many compassionate healers in it, we don't recommend chiropractors for primary care at any age. Chiropractors are not trained as broadly or as deeply as D.O.s and M.D.s, and they are not licensed to provide conventional care (drugs, surgery, in-hospital testing, etc.) when needed.

We have the following additional concerns about chiropractic care for children:

- Most chiropractors don't have special training in pediatric problems, which are very different from those of adults.

- Chiropractors aren't trained or licensed for comprehensive care, so they may not recognize serious illness and cannot prescribe drugs when needed.

- Chiropractic care can require frequent office visits. We recommend that parents carefully assess the need for further treatment after four or five sessions. We see no reason for healthy children to make the regular "maintenance" visits suggested by some chiropractors.

- A vocal element of the chiropractic profession has been very active in the debate against childhood immunizations, which we believe are essential.

- Some chiropractors make overzealous use of X-rays for diagnosis. We believe it's important to minimize both a child's exposure to X-rays and a parent's exposure to unnecessary costs.

- Many chiropractors make use of diagnostic tools such as applied kinesiology that are too unorthodox even for us.

Neither of us recommends chiropractic care for infants. We rarely recommend chiropractic therapy for children under age twelve. If you choose to go this route, ask your doctor for a referral to a chiropractor with whom he or she has a working relationship. We ourselves are more likely to refer children to a D.O. for gentle manipulation or cranial osteopathy because our training and approach to the care of children are so similar.

Massage

Isn't it great when something that feels so good is good for you, too? You might not realize it, but massage is more than just some "oohs" and "ahs" and a sense of well-being. As performed by professionals, massage can be used to stimulate, relax, or rehabilitate. According to studies done with children, therapeutic massage can improve colic, reduce levels of stress hormones in children with asthma, lower blood sugar levels in children with diabetes, reduce anxiety and depression, improve lung function in kids with cystic fibrosis, decrease restlessness in kids with ADD, and relieve sleep problems. Some research suggests massage therapy can even help premature babies gain weight more quickly. Not a bad record for something so simple and pleasant.

Some of the benefits of massage may be attributable to caring touch, but many come from actual physiological changes activated by the manipulation of skin, muscle, and joints. Touching someone in a caring way activates millions of sensory receptors on the skin, which can affect breathing, heart rate, and the production of hormones, immune cells, and other chemical transmitters. Far from being an indulgence, massage (either from a loved one or a professional) is an important way to maximize health.

Massage is a body therapy that can be enjoyed on a variety of levels, from amateur back rub to specialized professional massage therapy. Certification and licensure of massage therapists varies from state to state, but we recommend getting a referral from your child's doctor or the American Massage Therapy Association if your child needs massage for rehabilitation from injury, or has a condition that requires special care.

Parents make great massage therapists, too, starting right after baby is born. Brief periods of gentle massage can help babies sleep better, grow faster, bond sooner, and be less irritable. We teach infant massage techniques to new parents who are at a loss as to how to handle colicky or irritable babies. Massage soothes these babies and gives their parents a positive experience with them too.

more on . . .

INFANT MASSAGE

It's not tricky: Just mix one drop of lavender oil into a palmful of moisturizing cream or vegetable oil, then gently stroke your baby's body, uncurling clenched fingers, rubbing the feet in little circles. Use some pressure, so it doesn't feel like tickling. Do this at least once a day, especially at bedtime. Keep massage sessions short, no more than ten minutes at a time, as too much can overstimulate an infant. If you feel all thumbs around a new baby, you can take one of the popular baby massage classes being offered all over the country or purchase an instructional videotape. (See Resources.)

As your baby gets older, you can continue massage, maybe adding to your repertoire of massage moves by taking a class or learning through a book or video. Teach these techniques to your children as well, so that eventually everyone in the family knows how to give a back, shoulder, head, hand, or foot massage. Family massage is a handy stress-reduction technique, an easy way to help your children experience the sensation of truly relaxed muscles so they can better identify areas of tension, and a fine display of concern for others. Massage offers two-way satisfaction. Studies show that both the giver and the receiver of massage experience a reduction in feelings of anxiety and depression. And it's so simple. All you need is a firm but comfortable surface, a bottle of scented or unscented oil or lotion, and a body. A brief massage at bedtime is a great way to relax a child into sleep. And there's a two-way benefit, because you have to learn to let go of your own daily tension in order to do this properly.

We recommend a visit to a massage therapist for any member of the family who wants a real treat. In addition, professional massage may be therapeutic for children with muscle spasms and other musculoskeletal problems, and disorders such as recurrent infections (other than skin infections). In such cases, you may want to ask your doctor for a referral or ask around to find a therapist skilled in working with children.

A full professional massage generally takes place on a special padded table in a warm, relaxing environment. The child may be clothed if modesty is an issue, but it is preferable to have him undress to the underwear and be draped with a sheet, exposing only the areas being massaged at the time. The therapist will use oil or lotion to reduce friction. If it is scented, they may ask first if he likes the scent. Soft music is often played. Be sure to let him know it's OK to ask to have the music changed if it gets in the way of his enjoyment of the therapy. It is completely appropriate for a parent to stay in the room during a massage therapy session.

Energy Massage

There are several forms of massage that are aimed less at relaxing the muscles and more at releasing an unseen force the Chinese call *qi*, or *chi*. According to Chinese medicine, which we describe more fully in chapter 13, qi is the life force (energy) that travels freely through the body when we are healthy. Ill health comes from stagnation, blockage, excess, or loss of qi. Forms of massage designed to unlock energy and allow it to flow freely again include:

- *Acupressure* is a needleless version of Chinese acupuncture that relies on pressure from the fingers or thumbs on special points on the body to unblock qi. *Shiatsu* is a Japanese form of acupressure. *Tui na* is a unique form of Chinese medical massage therapy also meant to balance qi.
- *Reflexology* or *zone therapy* is a fairly modern modality based on the premise that areas on the feet, hands, and ears correspond directly to various parts of the body. Pressure applied—typically with the thumb—to a specific point is believed to open up energy blockages in the related area and help heal imbalance or illness there.

more on . . .

SWEDISH MASSAGE

The most common form of massage is Swedish massage, an adaptation of ancient Chinese techniques developed by a Swede in the nineteenth century. The five basic techniques of Swedish massage are:

1. *Stroking* (*effleurage*)–a gliding stroke with the palm, much like stroking a cat–is often used to begin or end a massage session.
2. *Kneading* (*petrissage*)–squeezing, pressing, and rolling the muscles using hands, thumbs, and fingers–is just like making bread.
3. *Friction*–deep circular or crosswise motions with the fingers or thumbs–relaxes "knots" in the muscles.
4. *Percussion* (*tapotement*)–gently striking the body with cupped hands, fingers, or the edge of the hand–may feel and sound like falling rain or a karate chop.
5. *Vibration*–gentle shaking, rolling action–feels not unlike a vibrator.

Other Forms of Bodywork

Bodywork techniques are all based on the idea that manipulation or movement of the body can free up restrictions imposed by habit or muscular tension that are affecting physical and emotional health. There are too many bodywork techniques for us to be able to discuss them all, so we will refer you to Mirka Knaster's excellent book *Discovering the Body's Wisdom* for more detail. Most of these other forms of bodywork are aimed at adults, who have had years to develop unhealthy patterns or injuries. We don't generally refer children for these therapies, except for children with scoliosis who may benefit from the Feldenkrais Method or the Alexander Technique.

Therapeutic Exercise

In the broad sense, exercise is a manual therapy too. It is well proven that exercise affects not just your bones and muscles but also your body systems and your emotions. Regular exercise boosts immunity; lowers the risk of cardiovascular disease, diabetes, osteoporosis, obesity, and certain cancers; and is a proven antidote to depression and anxiety.

In addition to informal methods of exercise, there are schools of what might be called *integrative exercise*, such as yoga and tai chi, which combine structured physical activity with a meditative element. We have already touched briefly on yoga in the previous chapter. Whereas yoga springs from India, tai chi is an ancient martial art form from China. Anyone who has ever lived in an area with a concentration of Chinese Americans has probably seen older people in the parks in the morning silently performing the slow sweeping movements of tai chi. These graceful movements are designed to facilitate the free flow of chi through the body, increase flexibility, and create balance in body and mind. The basic movements are simple, and they can easily be done by children.

CHAPTER 12

Herbs and Spices:

Botanical Medicine

Medicines made from the flowers, leaves, bark, roots, and other parts of plants have been the basis of medical care for millennia. About 30 percent of the prescription drugs on the market today (including important drugs for pain, heart disease, and cancer) were initially derived from plants. Conventional M.D.s in countries around the world prescribe herbal remedies as a matter of course. Pharmacies in those countries stock botanical medicines, and their staffs are able to offer informed advice to customers interested in herbal approaches. We are not so lucky here in the United States, where few conventional doctors or pharmacists are well trained in the use of botanicals. As a result, too many people rely on the advice of the clerks in health food stores, an approach we really don't recommend.

It is far safer to work in partnership with your doctor. In fact, we first began educating ourselves about the proper use of herbs because of our desire to provide better guidance to patients who were experimenting with botanicals. We wanted them to have solid information on the safest and most effective ways to use medicinal plants for themselves and their families. We are quite enthusiastic about the use of specific herbal remedies for adults, but we are more cautious about their use in children, because of the relative lack of data on the use of herbs in the young.

Until recently, Western medicine dismissed regional lore about botanical remedies as being backward, dangerous, and, well, dumb. Most Americans have lost—or never had—the familiarity with the use of local medicinal herbs that has been passed down through generations of local healers and "plant ladies." But the pendulum is swinging back, and sales of over-the-counter botanical remedies now top $4 billion a year in the United States.

This swing toward "natural" medicines comes with a few concerns. Contrary to myth, herbs are not necessarily safer than medications. Medicinal herbs may be less concentrated than conventional medicines, but they are still drugs, and they should be used with at least the same caution and respect given to their pharmaceutical cousins. "Natural" does not necessarily mean "safe." Some herbs are toxic with overdose, some interact adversely with prescription medication, and some are contaminated or made therapeutically worthless in processing. Parents need to treat herbal remedies with respect and not use an herbal remedy when the situation really calls for a visit to the doctor. Parents should also be wary of health care practitioners who regularly use herbs, vitamins, and supplements but dismiss the very real benefits of conventional medicine.

There is very little clinical data on the safety and efficacy of herbal remedies for children, but then, there hasn't been much on most prescription medicines for the under-twelve age group either. Despite the relative lack of medical research, we do think that there is a place for some botanical remedies in integrative pediatric care.

Using Herbs

We are not herbalists by trade or training, and your child's doctor is not likely to be one either. However, we did have unique in-depth training in the use of botanicals. Thanks to an explosion in research on botanical medicines in the past few years, and a significant amount of personal experience using plant medicines in our practices, we feel comfortable making some broad recommendations regarding the use of herbs in children. We predict that doctors and pharmacists will soon be more familiar with plant remedies and better able to educate parents about them. The United States Pharmacopoeia has set standards for the manufacture of some botanicals (look for the "USP" on the package), and the new FDA-mandated good manufacturing practices (GMPs) will soon be firmly in place.

We use select herbal remedies in treating our patients and our own children. We think that botanical remedies like the ones described in this chapter can safely be given to children in certain circumstances:

- ▶ To relieve symptoms or shorten the duration of self-limiting illnesses such as coughs, colds, car sickness, upset stomach, or the flu
- ▶ To shore up immune function for the short term, especially during the cold-and-flu season
- ▶ To help treat chronic conditions, such as eczema and recurrent ear or urinary tract infections
- ▶ To reduce the side effects of conventional medicine, such as nausea induced by chemotherapy
- ▶ As a tonic to strengthen or tone the organs and systems, especially after an illness. Western medicine relies on drugs with specific effects on specific conditions. In contrast, Eastern medicine places the highest value on tonic drugs/herbs that have more general effects and that work to enhance overall balance and increase resistance.

As integrative practitioners, we tend to turn to herbs as an alternative to over-the-counter medications and as a way to support the body's healing capacity. When properly used, herbs have a gentler action with fewer side effects, often at lower cost. Botanical medicines are available in a variety of forms, but we recommend standardized liquid or solid extracts, tinctures, or capsules of freeze-dried herbs (in that order) for oral use. (Remember, homeopathic medicines are made and used quite differently from botanicals, even though both may be based on plant substances.)

We prefer *single-plant products* from reputable manufacturers who guarantee that a certain percentage of the active or marker compounds of an herb will be present (a process called standardization). We look for *whole-herb products* rather than isolated factors from an herb because herbs have many constituent compounds; some produce the therapeutic effect and others act synergistically to enhance the benefit and reduce possible side effects. Truth is, we don't really have the research yet to know which compounds are truly extraneous. We do not recommend buying loose herbs or powdered herbs (with the exception of freeze-dried herbs) in capsules, as herbs deteriorate quickly when exposed to light and air.

The giant pharmaceutical companies now leaping into the botanicals market tend to treat herbs like chemical drugs, looking for the one active ingredient that they can extract, standardize, and package. There are both advantages and disadvantages to these products. They are more likely to be manufactured under safe, sanitary conditions and tested to assure that they contain exactly what they advertise. But some of the benefits seen when all the compounds in the herb are retained—such as reduced side effects, gentler action, and therapeutic synergy among the various constituents of the herb—may be lost.

There are a number of ways to give herbs to children. There are a growing number of better-tasting herbal remedies made specifically for kids. You can also add liquid extracts or tinctures to a strong-tasting juice like purple grape juice or to chocolate syrup. You can put them in a mug, add hot water to evaporate the alcohol, and serve when cooled with a little sweetener (avoid honey for kids under one). Capsules of freeze-dried herbs can be broken open and mixed into applesauce or used to make teas.

Using Botanicals Safely

The Food and Drug Administration classifies herbal remedies as "dietary supplements" rather than over-the-counter medicines, which means that their quality, their purity, and their advertising are regulated as foods and not as pharmaceuticals. Because the FDA hasn't had the funds or manpower to properly enforce even these regulations, consumers have been educating themselves about herbs and learning to identify manufacturers who voluntarily abide by recommendations for good manufacturing practices until the newly government-mandated guidelines take full effect.

If your child is seeing an integrative practitioner, you will have a knowledgeable partner with whom to discuss most any botanical remedy. However, many doctors are still learning about botanical medicine, or are closed to the idea. If you decide to use an herbal remedy on your child (or yourself) without the guidance of a professional, here are a few steps you should take first:

▶ *Do your research.* Make sure you know the correct diagnosis. Learn the scientific names of the best herbs for this condition, their specific uses, their possible side effects in good health or illness, and any potential interactions with food or drugs. (See Resources.)

▶ *Inform your doctor.* Your child's doctor needs to know about any herbs (or supplements) that your child is taking, even if that physician doesn't appear open to their use. It's the only way the doctor can protect your child from potential adverse interactions between those herbs and medication, and he or she may know of contraindications to the use of the herb of which you are not aware.

▶ *Be a careful shopper.* Know what you want before you go to the store. Product labels cannot by law tell you an herb's specific medical effects or its side effects, and you can't count on store clerks for unbiased and dependable information. Look for a standardized extract or tincture from a reputable manufacturer, and check that the expiration date has not passed. You want a fresh extract made with fresh herbs.

▶ *Use according to package directions for children.* Remember, there is still very little data on the use of herbs in children, so any suggested dosages are approximated. The general rule of thumb for children of average size is one half the adult dose for kids six to twelve, and one quarter the adult dose for kids two to six. Do not give children higher-than-recommended doses of an herb in the mistaken belief that more is better.

▶ *Be patient.* Don't expect an herb to work immediately. Most take days or weeks before results are seen.

▶ *Don't give children herbs for more than three weeks without follow-up.* Very little research has been done on the long-term effects of any herb on developing bodies. Most professional herbalists recommend taking an occasional break even from tonics, which are usually taken for weeks or months at a time.

more on . . .

IMPORTANT TERMS

Tonic. A tonic herb such as astragalus or maitake mushroom is taken regularly for the generalized effect of strengthening and toning the body. It helps the body respond better to physical and emotional stress, and normalizes function (both excess and deficiency).

Tincture. The fluid that is pressed or filtered out after an herb has been soaked in alcohol and/or water or other solvent mixtures to separate out the medicinal agents.

Extract. In liquid form, a more concentrated tincture that contains less alcohol and more plant material. Solid extracts—liquid extracts with the solvents removed—are more stable and more concentrated than liquid extracts.

Standardized extract. An herb that has been distilled and processed to contain certain levels of the active compound, or a marker compound if the active agent is unknown. Standardized extracts may be more expensive, but they offer the best assurance of a consistent, quality product, because levels of the active compounds in medicinal plants can vary tremendously depending on individual plant makeup and growing, harvesting, and storage conditions.

Freeze-dried extracts. Liquid extracts that have had their solvents removed through flash evaporation. These encapsulated products are more stable than air-dried extracts and herbs.

Herb teas. Single herbs or herb blends dried and sold loose or in tea bags to be steeped in hot water and served warm or cold. Teas are weakened by exposure to air, light, and moisture, so use only teas packed either in opaque, resealable bags or in sealed single servings.

Ground or powdered herbs in capsules. Not recommended due to greater exposure to air, heat, light, and moisture during processing and storage.

Loose or bulk herbs. Not recommended, as they are usually the least active and most unstable form.

▶ *Avoid using more than one herb at a time without professional guidance.* We don't yet know enough about herb-herb interactions, especially in children.

▶ *Be careful using herbs in children under two years of age.* The only herbs we regularly use orally in children this age are chamomile or peppermint teas. We make short-term use of topical calendula for diaper rash, and we occasionally employ echinacea or garlic for colds in children older than 15 months.

▶ *Watch for allergic reactions.* Discontinue the herb and contact your child's doctor if symptoms such as skin rash, wheezing, vomiting, tummy ache, or nausea develop.

▶ *Stop using any herbs 10 to 14 days before any surgical procedure.* Some herbs—especially ginger and garlic—can increase bleeding at such times.

TIP: You needn't worry about giving your children alcohol-based botanicals, since a child really gets only a few drops of alcohol from a dose of a liquid extract or tincture. Much of the alcohol will evaporate if the extract or tincture is served in a warm drink. Nonalcoholic vinegar- or glycerin-based extracts just aren't as effective in our experience.

Buying Botanical Medicines

Herbal products are easily available in the marketplace, and their claims may be quite extravagant, so allow us to offer some guidance. Start with some research of your own and consultation with your child's doctor to determine the herb needed. Visit a trusted Web site (see Resources) that offers information on the quality of various herbal products by brand. In addition:

▶ Look for products from reputable companies using good manufacturing practices.

▶ Look for standardized extracts for a better guarantee that the product will contain a specified amount of an active or marker compound.

- Look for products that contain the same species (Latin name) and the same parts of the plant used in the scientific medical research you have found.

- Look for products that use fresh herbs. Check the expiration date to make sure the product is fresh too.

- Look for organic products when possible.

- Look for the letters NF or USP to indicate the product meets standards set by the United States Pharmacopoeia.

- Look for single-herb products rather than combinations.

- Check the dosage. Two brands may charge the same dollar amount for 60 capsules, but if the daily dosage is 500 mg and the capsules in one bottle are 100 mg and the capsules in the other are 250 mg, the second bottle is obviously the better buy.

The Herbal Medicine Chest

The herbs described below are the ones we have found to be most helpful with children's conditions. Please see the appropriate chapters in Section III for dosages and other information for specific conditions. We've already gone over general herb safety issues, so we've only included more specific concerns below:

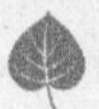

Aloe (*Aloe vera*). Every kitchen should have an easy-to-grow, undemanding aloe plant in a pot on the windowsill. Then if little (or big) fingers get burned, all you have to do is slice off a little piece of this succulent tropical plant and apply the gel inside.

Use: Aloe can be used for kitchen burns, sunburn, canker sores, insect bites, psoriasis, and minor abrasions.

Form: Apply either a store-bought pure-aloe gel, or the sticky, soothing gel found inside the middle portion of the aloe leaf to the burn.

Concerns: Don't use aloe on surgical wounds, as there are some concerns it may actually slow down the healing process. Don't take aloe internally, as it occasionally causes gastrointestinal cramping.

Astragalus (*Astragalus membranaceus*). Astragalus, or *huangqi*, is a member of the pea family whose sweet-tasting root is commonly used in Traditional Chinese Medicine to enhance immunity and prevent disease. Astragalus appears to increase the production of white blood cells and immune mediators such as interferon.

Use: Astragalus is used to help regain strength after flu; to build resistance in kids who have been suffering recurrent colds, flu, or bronchitis; and to support immune function during chemotherapy. It can also be taken daily as a tonic to prevent upper respiratory infections, ear infections, or the flu.

Form: Take as a tincture or as a liquid or solid standardized extract.

Dosage: As a tonic, take 4 to 8 drops of liquid standardized extract or tincture every twelve hours for kids aged two to six. Take 8 to 15 drops, or 250 to 500 mg, of standardized solid extract in capsules every twelve hours for kids six to twelve years old.

Concerns: As far as we know, there are no cautions for this herb, though some practitioners suggest taking a week off every month.

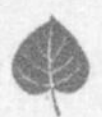

Calendula (*Calendula officinalis*). Compounds in the edible flowers of this relative of the garden marigold act as an antiseptic and an anti-inflammatory.

Use: Calendula can be used for skin problems like abrasions, burns, diaper rashes, and eczema.

Form: Can be found as a lotion, gel, or cream.

Concerns: May occasionally worsen skin irritation.

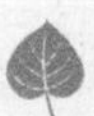

Chamomile (either German, *Matricaria recutita*, or Roman, *Anthemis nobilis*). The daisylike flowers of this fragrant, low-growing plant have been used as a sedative and digestive aid for centuries.

Use: Chamomile is used for the treatment of colic, anxiety, teething, upset stomach, or difficulties falling asleep.

Form: Drink warm or cool fresh tea steeped ten to fifteen minutes and diluted to taste.

Buying tips: Buy tea bags in sealed single packets for freshness.

Concerns: It's unlikely, but children who are severely allergic to ragweed may be allergic to chamomile, a member of the same plant family. Pregnant moms should not drink chamomile tea, as the herb can cause uterine contractions.

Echinacea (*Echinacea purpurea, angustifolia,* and *pallida*). The roots, leaves, flowers, seeds, and juice of various species of the beautiful purple coneflower appear to stimulate the immune system.

Use: When taken at the first sign of illness, echinacea may prevent the development of upper respiratory tract infections such as colds and flu or may shorten the duration of these illnesses. May also be helpful for ear infections, bladder infections, and perhaps as supportive therapy for recurrent vaginal yeast infections, but research is scant.

Form: Take as a standardized liquid or solid extract or as a tincture. (Many products come combined with goldenseal [*Hydrastis canadensis*], but the second herb isn't necessary.)

Buying tips: Because most research has been done on the aboveground parts of *Echinacea purpurea*, that is the species we recommend, alone or combined with the roots of *E. angustifolia* (another well-researched extract). The most therapeutically effective echinacea liquid extracts and tinctures cause a tingling or numbing sensation on the tongue.

Concerns: There is a theoretical concern about the use of echinacea for children with autoimmune disorders or HIV or for children with an allergy to plants in the daisy family.

Elderberry (*Sambucus nigra*). The berry of the European black elder contains compounds that inhibit multiple strains of flu virus from reproducing in the body.

Use: Elderberry can be used to reduce the duration or intensity of the flu. Dr. D has also found that it often shortens the severity and duration of a cold.

Form: Take as a standardized liquid extract.

Concerns: It should *not* be considered an alternative to the flu vaccine.

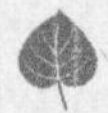

Garlic (*Allium sativum*). This familiar kitchen herb, and its relative the onion (*Allium cepa*), provide sulfur-containing compounds that appear to lower blood pressure, decrease cholesterol, fight disease-causing microbes, and improve immune function.

Use: Garlic can be used to help stave off upper respiratory and perhaps fungal infections.

Form: Give your kids lots of garlic in their food. Just chop garlic, let it rest for a few minutes to develop the most beneficial compounds, and use raw or lightly cooked. For kids who don't like the taste or smell, standardized deodorized garlic extracts are available in solid or liquid form.

Concerns: Garlic or onion intake by a breast-feeding mother may cause stomach upset in sensitive infants, though there is conflicting evidence that some babies feed better when nursing moms eat these herbs. They may interact with some prescription medications.

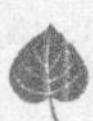

Ginger (*Zingiber officinale*). Ginger is familiar to us all as an ingredient in ginger ale, gingersnaps, and some great Chinese food. This root has also long been used in Traditional Chinese Medicine as an anti-inflammatory and to relieve nausea.

Use: Ginger is used to treat motion sickness, nausea, tummy aches, migraines, and inflammatory conditions such as juvenile rheumatoid arthritis.

Form: Ginger can be eaten as a food or candy (watch out, though, it's hot!), grated or sliced thinly and used to make a tea with honey, or taken as a liquid or freeze-dried extract.

Concerns: Theoretically, it could increase the risk of bleeding.

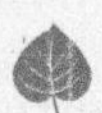

Green tea (*Camellia sinensis*). Green tea is simply a less-processed version of the familiar dark brown tea. The potential health benefits of green tea are a hot research topic these days, with studies suggesting that the antioxidants and other healthful compounds in green tea can lower cholesterol, reduce the risk of heart disease and cancer, protect skin, prevent cavities, and fight bacteria.

Use: Introduce your children to the taste of green tea while they are young so they can reap its potential long-term benefits.

Form: Take as loose or bagged green tea steeped in hot but not boiling water for just a few minutes. Can also be served iced. Organic versions can be found.

Concerns: Infants should not be given green tea, as there have been reports that it may interfere with their absorption of iron. Green tea contains about as much caffeine as a cola drink, and a quarter to an eighth the caffeine of coffee (depending on your blend). While decaffeinated brands are available, we prefer you use caffeinated forms, but drink only the second or third steeping, which contains much less caffeine.

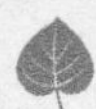

Peppermint (*Mentha piperita*). The lush, green, spreading herb peppermint has a long history of safe use as a digestive aid.

Use: Peppermint can be used to soothe upset tummy or colic in little ones or to treat irritable bowel syndrome (IBS) in older children.

Form: Take as fresh tea cooled to lukewarm, or for IBS, as enteric-coated capsules that insure the peppermint oil will not be released until it reaches the intestines.

Buying tips: Make sure to buy single, sealed tea bags or the enteric-coated capsules.

Concerns: Use only enteric-coated forms of the oil. Children with reflux should avoid *any* form of peppermint, as it relaxes the sphincter between stomach and esophagus and can worsen their symptoms.

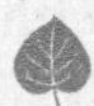

Slippery Elm (*Ulmus rubra*). The inner bark of slippery elm is what herbalists call a demulcent, that is, it soothes mucous membranes.

Use: Slippery elm can be used for sore throats, coughs, and intestinal upsets.

Form: Take as lozenges, or as a tea of 1 or 2 teaspoons of slippery elm powder in hot water for upper respiratory problems. Take as a thin gruel of the powder mixed with warm water or milk for gastrointestinal problems.

Concerns: Avoid whole bark products, as they may slow absorption of other medications.

We'd also like to mention one more "herb" that might not ordinarily come to mind. Medicinal mushrooms—especially reishi (*Ganoderma lucidum*), shiitake (*Lentinus elodes*), and maitake (*Grifola frondosa*)—have been eaten in Asia for centuries as a way to boost the immune system. Today they are also an important complement to conventional cancer treatment in Japan and China, and may help lower cholesterol levels as well. These mushrooms are best cooked and eaten as foods or made into teas, but they are also available as extracts (look for those labeled aflatoxin-free). Dr. D frequently gives his patients a special extract of maitake mushroom for fighting upper respiratory infections and flu.

Essential Oils

In addition to these oral and topical uses of medicinal plants, there is a whole school of therapy based on the use of essential plant oils to influence physical and emotional well-being. You are probably familiar with beauty products, room fragrances, and candles that employ *aromatherapy* but may not have realized that essential oils of lavender, orange, vanilla, and other plants have therapeutic uses as well. We use aromatherapy diffusers in our offices to create a more relaxed and welcoming atmosphere. These essential oils are finding their way into hospitals (scents are used to relax people having medical procedures such as magnetic resonance imaging), massage-therapy offices, and other therapeutic locations especially because of their ability to influence mood.

Essential oils—highly concentrated plant extracts—are very strong and potentially toxic, so if they are to be used with children, special care must be taken to avoid oral use (an exception is made for enteric-coated peppermint oil for children over 44 pounds) or use of the undiluted oil directly on a child's skin. Never apply essential oils in or around the nose, mouth, or eyes of a child. Instead confine their use to the areas of chest and back. Keep them where children cannot reach them, as drinking them can be lethal. When buying an essential oil, make sure to get pure products and not synthetic scents. For instance, don't be fooled into buying lavendin (a synthetic) rather than oil of lavender.

TWELVE USEFUL HERBS FOR CHILDREN

Echinacea for colds and perhaps flu

Astragalus as a tonic, especially after or to prevent recurrent respiratory illness

Ginger for nausea, tummy troubles, and inflammation

Garlic for mild infections

Elderberry for flu

Chamomile for colic, teething, anxiety, sleeplessness

Peppermint for tummy troubles

Slippery elm for sore throat, tummy troubles

Green tea for general good health

Calendula for diaper rash and other skin problems

Aloe for burns

Eucalyptus for congestion (aromatherapy)

We are not experts on the use of essential oils but have dabbled with some of the more common agents and modes of delivery. We rarely use more than one or two drops of an essential oil at a time. When an essential oil is to be used on a child's skin, it should always be well diluted in lotion or a vegetable or nut "carrier" oil such as almond or olive oil. With essential oils, less is more. You really only need one drop of an oil on a child's blanket or pillow, one drop in a warm bath, one or two drops in a handful of carrier oil or lotion, or a few drops in a diffuser (which warms and spreads the scent with no physical contact with the oil). The essential oils we are most comfortable using with children are the following:

Lavender (*Lavendula angustifolia*). Studies have found lavender oil to have both antiseptic and sedative properties. We use it mostly for relaxation—on a blanket, in bath water, in massage oil, or through a diffuser. Vanilla has a similar relaxing effect for some people. In France, bunches or bags of lavender flowers are often hung near a child's cot to promote restful sleep. It should not be used repeatedly on the skin until concerns over its estrogenic properties have been resolved.

Eucalyptus (*Eucalyptus radiata*). The leaves of this tree from Australia contain aromatic oils that fight congestion and bacteria. We recommend 1 or 2 drops of essential oil of eucalyptus in a cup of vegetable oil as a rub for a congested chest. A single drop of eucalyptus oil can also be put on a corner of a child's blanket to help unstuff a stuffy nose. Eucalyptus oil is poisonous, so keep it—and all essential oils—out of the reach of children.

Tea tree (*Melaleuca alternifolia*). We recommend it in a diluted form as a natural antiseptic for cuts, scrapes, insect bites, and acne. We also use it diluted as a topical antifungal for athlete's foot and ringworm and carefully apply it undiluted on fungal nails or, per Dr. D, directly on viral warts (*Molluscum contagiosum*). Be cautious with use, as tea tree oil is strong and can cause a rash in sensitive people.

CHAPTER 13

Other Alternatives:

Chinese, Homeopathic, and Energy Medicines

In this chapter we want to tell you about three other forms of complementary and alternative medicine that we sometimes find useful—traditional Chinese medicine (TCM), homeopathy, and energy medicine. Though they come from different sources, they share a belief that subtle energies in the body can influence health.

As integrative doctors, we borrow extensively from the philosophy of TCM and regularly refer patients to its practitioners. We are also believers in the potential therapeutic benefits to be found in the gentle, compassionate practice of energy healing in the right hands. We are intrigued by reports of the usefulness of homeopathy in certain circumstances, and on occasion make clinical use of certain homeopathic remedies, but only rarely refer patients for constitutional evaluation and treatment. There are, of course, other complete systems of health care deserving of our attention, including ayurveda, naturopathy, and Tibetan medicine, but we don't address them here because our experience with them is limited.

Chinese Medicine

You're probably familiar with the Oriental medical practice of acupuncture, but you may not realize that acupuncture is just one of five major branches of a complex system of medicine that also encompasses herbal treatments, medicinal nutrition, therapeutic massage, and meditative exercise. Studies published in Western medical journals have reported that various forms of traditional Chinese medicine (TCM) may be useful for pain, asthma, ear infections, headache, insomnia, eczema, irritable bowel syndrome, balance problems, high blood pressure, sports injuries, and chemotherapy-induced nausea. There is a vast amount of clinical evidence published in Chinese medical literature for other uses as well.

We ourselves are not practitioners of TCM, but we are fortunate to have received extensive training in it. We regularly refer patients to practitioners of TCM to get therapy for certain acute conditions and for many chronic conditions for which Western medicine has no cure or clear treatment. Although we find the philosophy behind Chinese medicine appealing, we don't begin to understand how it works. We only know that it frequently gets results in cases that have stymied Western medical specialists.

What Is Chinese Medicine?

Over the past few millennia the Chinese have developed a system of medicine quite unlike our own. While Western doctors were still bleeding, purging, and otherwise mishandling the sick, the Chinese already possessed a sophisticated medical philosophy and numerous noninvasive therapies that had been tested over generations. We use the term *medical philosophy* because to the Chinese, healing was part and parcel of their Taoist philosophy of wholeness and balance. The basis of both healing practice and spiritual practice was the concept of qi or chi (pronounced *chee*), the invisible life force or flow of vital energy that circulates throughout the universe, and permeates the human body. In a healthy person, qi flows unimpeded. However, when qi is blocked, or when it stagnates in one area, an imbalance is created that manifests as illness. The purpose of Chinese medicine is to locate and release these obstructions, and restore good health by moving qi into areas where it is lacking.

more on . . .

YIN AND YANG

The rock-bottom foundation of TCM is the principle of yin and yang, universal forces of energy that must be in balance for physical and social health. The balance between yin and yang is dynamic. It can vary by time of day, physical condition, energetic excesses or deficiencies, diet, stage of life, etc. We all have both yin and yang within us, even though yin is described as "female" and yang as "male." Yin is considered to be moist, cold, dark, passive, material, and nourishing. Yang is considered to be dry, hot, light, active, energetic, and transforming. The best description we have seen of this duality comes from the book *Between Heaven and Earth: A Guide to Chinese Medicine*. "If *Yin* is a noun, then *Yang* is a verb, and life is a complete sentence."

The practitioner of TCM compares himself to a gardener (a telling difference from the Western doctor-as-warrior or doctor-as-mechanic metaphors) whose goal is to tend so well to all the aspects of the patient that the individual can meet any challenges to his health. Treatment is based not just on physical symptoms but also on the person's emotional and energetic state, as well as his relationship with his physical and social environment. While sometimes the goal is just to relieve symptoms, more frequently the goal is to balance and strengthen the body so that healing can take place.

The basic principles and modalities of Chinese medicine have been adapted over the centuries to reflect various schools of thought and national differences. Today the Chinese health system also offers the techniques of conventional Western medicine, in much the same way as we in the West have been adapting traditional Chinese therapies into our own medical practice. For instance, herbs integral to Chinese medicine, such as ginger, ginseng, and licorice, are now mainstays of Western herbal medicine too. Acupuncture is now practiced in the United States not only by those trained at colleges of acupuncture and Oriental medicine here and in China but also by M.D.s trained in a more Westernized version.

TCM is a complete system of medicine, although it is more commonly used in the United States as a complement to conventional medicine. Based on the ideal of harmony and balance, TCM teaches that a truly healthy person needs to be in harmony within body, family, community, and universe. We find this very poetic approach to health especially appealing as it underscores the importance of integration of mind and body and interconnection with our neighbors and our surroundings. However, the very poetics of TCM may make it difficult for Western minds to wrap around it. We are not accustomed to medical practitioners who talk about yin and yang, the Three Treasures, the Five Elements, the Eight Principles, or an invisible organ like the Triple Burner.

TCM offers individualized treatment that takes into account the full person and that person's role in family and community, looking very closely at the underlying emotional or energetic causes for symptoms, assessing the general state of health, and choosing from a wide variety of possible remedies. That is why, unlike in Western medicine, two people with the same diagnosis—indigestion, for example—may well be given different treatments. And that is why, unlike in Western medicine, two people with different symptoms may well be given the same treatment, if a practitioner feels the same underlying imbalance is at work in both cases.

Visiting a Practitioner of Chinese Medicine

As you can imagine, a visit to a practitioner of TCM is very different from a visit to an M.D. The TCM practitioner will take a thorough medical history and perform a specialized physical examination, but that's where the resemblance ends. A doctor of Chinese medicine may ask whether your child is thirsty, where and how she sweats, how connected she feels to your family, and other unusual questions. Some of the physical symptoms attended to (such as how your child smells) will be atypical as well. The doctor will typically feel for not just one pulse in an older child's wrist, but three—and at two different depths, for a total of six pulses at each wrist—to determine the state of the various organs. In infants and younger children, the veins at the base of each index finger may be examined, as will the appearance of the tongue. The child's body will be palpated at acupuncture and other points, looking for tender areas. The intention is to evaluate the life force in your child's body—how it is moving, where it is blocked, and where it is stagnant. Treatment may involve some form of acupuncture or massage to normalize or enhance the flow of qi, and/or a combination of herbs to address systemic excesses or deficiencies.

Ideally, you can get a referral to a practitioner of Chinese medicine from your child's doctor. If that's not possible, look for a practitioner who uses the true Eastern-philosophy-based approach and has had the extensive training and clinical experience required for an O.M.D. (Oriental medical doctor), an M.Ac.O.M. (a three-year master's degree in acupuncture and Oriental medicine), or L.Ac. (licensed acupuncturist). He or she should have either trained in China or graduated from three- to four-year training at an accredited college of Chinese medicine. Try to find a practitioner who is certified by the National Commission for the Certification of Acupuncturists and Oriental Medicine (NCCAOM). (See Resources.) Your insurance may cover these health care professionals, especially if your doctor refers you.

We believe that children should get their primary care from an M.D. or a D.O. trained to recognize the warning signs of serious medical illness. However, we do think Chinese medicine can be very useful for preventive care or for complementary treatment of some short- and long-term conditions. Just be sure your child's pediatrician is aware of your visits to the acupuncturist or O.M.D., and that the TCM practitioner is aware of any conventional medications your child is taking. A child should not stop important drugs, such as those for asthma or arthritis, while undergoing TCM treatment, although the treatments may eventually enable your child's doctor to reduce the drug dosage. Be very cautious with the use of Chinese medicinal herbs in children.

The Five Branches of TCM

Acupuncture

This is the form of TCM we most frequently recommend and that people in the United States are most likely to use. There are a number of systems of acupuncture being practiced, but they are all based on the idea that qi flows through invisible meridians, or channels, that form the energy distribution network of the body. A skilled practitioner is able to either activate or inhibit qi in organs associated with an acupuncture point by inserting very fine, fresh needles into the body at that point and letting them rest there for a period of time. Sometimes the needles are intermittently turned by hand or even attached to a low electrical current. This does not feel like an injection. There may be no discomfort at all besides a quick "tug," or a brief stinging sensation when a needle is inserted. Once the needles are inserted, many people report a sense of well-being and relaxation, to the point of falling asleep fully clothed on the treatment table.

Traditional Chinese acupuncture works with the whole body. There are forms developed in other countries that work only on points in the ear, hand, foot, or scalp to address issues in the whole body. In this country we also have a hybrid form of acupuncture practiced by many medical doctors that is called medical acupuncture. Medical acupuncture typically uses certain points identified as being associated with specific conventional Western diagnoses, rather than looking at the whole person and customizing treatment. Even though it appears to offer symptomatic relief to many patients, our preference remains the TCM approach.

Some practitioners of Chinese medicine work only on children above the age of seven, believing that the qi of younger children is too changeable. Others choose to use smaller and finer needles inserted more shallowly and for shorter lengths of time when working with younger children, in deference to their smaller size and more immature systems. The idea is just to give the body a subtle push that allows it to adjust itself.

Most children don't actually seem to mind acupuncture needles. If your child squawks at the idea, you might consider a form of needleless acupuncture, such as needleless electroacupuncture, magnet acupuncture, moxibustion (use of heat over acupuncture points), acupressure, or laser acupuncture, or Japanese systems of needleless pediatric acupuncture, such as *toyo hari* or *Shonishin*, which use special tools to stroke or tap acupuncture points.

more on . . .

HOW ACUPUNCTURE MAY WORK

Although there are studies and a great deal of anecdotal evidence that acupuncture can be effective for a number of conditions in children and adults, no one really knows how it works from a Western perspective. It's clearly not just a placebo effect. It appears that acupuncture can stimulate the production of pituitary hormones called endorphins that can relieve pain and affect the brain's production of neurotransmitters and other chemicals as well. In recent neuro-imaging studies, stimulating acupuncture points distant from the head that are traditionally associated with the eye and ear was seen to affect the portions of the brain that control vision and hearing.

We're fine with parents who take their children to an acupuncturist for problems such as colds, sinusitis, chronic cough, ear infections, asthma, headaches, dental pain, or constipation/diarrhea, provided significant illness has been excluded. We frequently refer patients for acupuncture for headaches, nausea, depression, and anxiety. A child whose system appears to be out of balance (from chronic illness or severe stress, for example) is also a good candidate for acupuncture.

Of course, you can't do acupuncture on your children at home, which is why acupressure is such a useful tool for parents and kids. Acupressure moves qi by applying firm pressure rather than needles to acupuncture points. There is currently less supportive data for acupressure, but it has been used successfully to treat headache, dental pain, nasal congestion, asthma, fatigue, stomach problems, and the nausea of seasickness or chemotherapy, as well as to maintain general good health. Your TCM practitioner can teach you several useful points and how to correctly apply pressure over them.

Chinese Medical Massage

Tui na (also called *tuina* or "pushing and pulling") uses soft-tissue massage and acupressure techniques to move qi in the body of a (usually clothed) patient. Tui na is often offered as a form of needleless acupuncture for children. The hand movements involved are very detailed and precise, so it would best to look for a practitioner with thorough training and much clinical experience.

Chinese Herbs

TCM makes extensive use of a wide array of plant, animal, and mineral substances, which are all categorized as herbal remedies. A true Chinese pharmacy is a fascinating place, loaded with boxes, jars, and drawers full of interesting things that have been used over the course of three thousand years to treat specific excesses or deficits in the organs and their systems. Western researchers are just beginning to look more closely at Chinese herbal formulas, and recent articles in major medical journals have reported some of them to be quite effective in the treatment of conditions such as irritable bowel syndrome, heart disease, and eczema.

more on . . .

USING CHINESE MEDICINAL HERBS SAFELY

For safety's sake, use fresh loose herbs only if they have been prescribed and provided by a reputable, licensed practitioner. When using preformulated tablets, capsules, pellets, or liquid extracts, buy only products made by reputable American companies, which have been prescribed and/or dispensed by your practitioner. We strongly advise against buying any Chinese patent remedies you find in Chinese markets or grocery stores. These products are frequently adulterated with prescription drugs, heavy metals, and other unwanted substances.

In keeping with the principles of harmony and balance, herbs are always given in combination, rather than singly. An herbal prescription may include both major herbs that deal directly with the problem and minor ones that work synergistically with them and prevent side effects. Traditionally these herbs are combined and then cooked or made into a tea. Since many of these teas taste and smell awful, common herbal combinations are also available in tablets, capsules, pellets, or liquid extracts.

Many Chinese herbal remedies have been safely used in small doses in children for generations, so they are probably safe if the herbs have been properly identified and freshly collected, if they have been safely stored and processed, and if they are correctly prescribed. These are a lot of "ifs." The appropriate use of Chinese medicinal herbs is a specialty unto itself, and because of our inexperience in this realm we remain very cautious about Chinese herbology with children. We generally recommend only the select use of specific Asian herbs, like ginger or astragalus, and then as single remedies rather than as parts of a compound remedy.

Exercise/Meditation

Chinese medicine makes use of age-old exercises combining physical action and meditation to promote the proper flow of qi through the body. These disciplines are considered to be "internal" martial arts because of the meditative component, and they are recommended for self-care to maintain good health and prevent illness. The most familiar to Westerners is tai chi. The gentle and slow-moving exercises of tai chi are very useful for improving balance and flexibility and for reducing stress. Each exercise has a fascinating name—such as Waving Hands in the Clouds and White Crane Spreads Its Wings—that provides an image of how the movement should be done. Children may enjoy tai chi, especially when done with their parents.

Qigong (sometimes seen as *chi gong*) encompasses many forms of exercise and meditation, as well as a therapeutic practice. Exercises vary from the nearly passive to the dynamic, so some form of qigong can be done even by the bedridden. Medical qigong as practiced traditionally in China employs these exercises both for preventive health care and for complementary therapy for chronic conditions. In China there are also expert practitioners of qigong who are apparently able to transmit their strong qi to others to stimulate healing. While we have heard some fascinating stories about how this form of energy healing is used in traditional Chinese hospitals, the possibilities for fraud or misrepresentation of skills and training seem too great here in the United States, where experts are few and far between. That's why we'll stick with recommending qigong solely for self-care and maintenance of general good health.

Medicinal Foods

In traditional Chinese medicine most foods are either yin or yang and can thus be used to balance an excess or deficiency of these elements in the body. Foods are considered to be able to heat or cool, increase moisture or dryness, build qi and blood, normalize function, and restore proper digestion. For instance, an O.M.D. might suggest that a person with nausea eat some warming ginger to dispel the cold in his system. Someone who feels tired and low on energy might be advised to eat foods such as yams and dates that boost qi. In China there are even restaurants that combine diagnosis with food, cooking dishes to order with ingredients that address a person's specific health problems! Our mothers, on the other hand, are firmly convinced that chicken soup or tea and crackers will cure anything that ails us.

Homeopathic Medicine

Homeopathy was once the most popular form of medical care in the United States. In the late 1880s there were twenty-two colleges of medicine and more than a hundred hospitals based on the principles of homeopathy developed by German physician Samuel Hahnemann. With the rise of allopathic medicine in the twentieth century, homeopathy was pushed to the fringes here. Yet many conventional physicians in Great Britain, Germany, France, India, and some parts of South America are still trained in homeopathic medicine and prescribe homeopathic remedies as a matter of course. Now Americans are reacquainting themselves with this gentle alternative medical system, and the market for homeopathic remedies for self-care is booming, especially for children.

What Is Homeopathy?

Homeopathic medicine is based on three principles, one of which conventional doctors can easily embrace, one that gives them some discomfort, and one they find hard to swallow:

1. The unique nature of a person makes individualization of therapy mandatory for clinical success.

2. Substances that cause certain symptoms in healthy people can cure those same symptoms in sick people ("like cures like"). Symptoms are seen as the body's attempt to heal, so remedies are intended to support this healing.

3. The most dilute substances may have the strongest effects. The most potent remedies are those that have been diluted and vigorously shaken ("succussed") the most times—so many times, in fact, that the strongest remedies may not even have a complete molecule of the therapeutic substance left in them.

The homeopathic approach runs counter to our conventional allopathic practice of using strong medicines that suppress symptoms, so it raises a lot of questions. How can sick people with fever and chills be cured by a medicine that gives healthy people fever and chills? How can little sugar pills that may contain less than a molecule of the allegedly therapeutic agent have any effect? How can pills made from odd and sometimes toxic substances such as squid ink, daisies, arsenic, and table salt do any good, let alone be safe?

We looked at homeopathic medicine with a pretty jaundiced eye at first too. But we kept hearing good reports from patients who were using homeopathic remedies to nip influenza in the bud, treat ear infections, ease teething pain, and take the "owie" out of bee stings. Now we no longer dismiss homeopathy as an oddball practice. Even though we cannot explain how it works, it does work in select circumstances. Most conventional Western medical authorities say any positive results seen with homeopathy are due to a placebo effect (but some studies cast doubt on that theory).

We are still just getting acquainted with the homeopathic approach, but we feel comfortable recommending homeopathy to parents to use on their children for first aid and minor, self-limiting illnesses because the remedies are safe, inexpensive, and—when used properly—often appear to be of benefit. Rarely, we refer parents of children with chronic illnesses (such as asthma, recurrent ear infections, anxiety, or attention deficit disorder) that might benefit from an in-depth homeopathic evaluation and stronger remedies to a medical, osteopathic, or naturopathic physician who is board certified in classical homeopathy. We do not recommend homeopathic medicine for acute, life-threatening illness or in any circumstance where conventional medical intervention is clearly warranted.

Visiting a Homeopath

Homeopathic practitioners—much like practitioners of osteopathy, chiropractic, and Chinese medicine—believe that there is a subtle energy that is the foundation of good health. Symptoms are seen as the body's attempts to heal itself, and this process is reinforced by medications that produce the same symptoms. This is a radically different perspective from conventional Western medicine, which is focused on getting rid of symptoms.

A "classical" homeopath relies on the interview more than on physical examination or laboratory testing. A first visit usually lasts an hour and a half to two hours (subsequent visits are much shorter). During that time, a homeopath will listen carefully and ask many questions, some of which might seem off-the-wall. The patient will not only be asked to describe the symptoms that brought him or her to the office, but he also might be asked about the influences upon him at the time he became sick, whether he is currently cranky or worried or frightened, whether he feels better when hot or when cold, what foods he craves or cannot bear, and so on. The object of this interview is to assemble a constitutional profile of a patient that includes his or her unique combination of physical symptoms, personality, likes and dislikes, and mental and emotional state. On the basis of this unique profile, the homeopath chooses the one constitutional remedy that will bring this patient back into physical and emotional balance. Such a remedy is expected to cure not only the presenting problem but all other symptoms as well. If it does not show effect within five weeks, another remedy may be prescribed.

Classical homeopaths as well as many conventional medical practitioners may also do what is called *clinical* or *acute prescribing*, in which the focus is less on correcting your child's constitutional imbalances than treating the current problem that has brought the child to the office. In this case, the practitioner examines the way this particular cold, say, affects this particular child physically and emotionally in order to determine which of the single cold remedies is best suited to his or her symptoms. The remedy will be less potent and taken more frequently than a constitutional remedy, should work more quickly, and will not be expected to treat anything but the presenting problem.

We have heard anecdotal evidence of excellent results from constitutional and acute remedies prescribed by homeopaths. We recommend you look for an experienced health practitioner who is board certified in homeopathy, has at least five hundred to one thousand hours of training, and is accustomed to working with children. There are only a few thousand M.D.s, osteopaths, naturopaths, and other health professionals in this country who are well trained in homeopathic medicine (see Resources), so there may not be one in your area. However, because this form of medicine relies so strongly on the interview, telephone consultations with distant practitioners are also a possibility. Do not follow the recommendations of any practitioner who advises the use of homeopathic remedies in place of vaccines.

more on . . .

HOW HOMEOPATHY MAY WORK

There are all sorts of theories as to how homeopathy might work, the acceptance of which generally depends on a willingness to suspend current medical beliefs. Some advocates of homeopathy suggest that certain steps in the preparation of a highly dilute homeopathic remedy make available the inherent "vital energy" of the active substance, perhaps by imprinting the remedy with the "memory" of this agent. (See why homeopathy is hard for Western science to swallow?) If homeopathy is indeed a form of energy medicine as some hypothesize, Western medicine may need to change its current understanding of healing before we even have the concepts and tools to figure out how homeopathy works. However, in the case of homeopathy we think it may be less important to ask, "Does it make sense?" than, "Does it work?" And it's only fair to point out that we don't understand how many conventional treatments work either.

Using Homeopathic Remedies for Self-Care

Homeopathic remedies are made from a wide variety of substances found in nature. *Allium cepa*, a common remedy for the weeping eyes and runny nose of colds, is made from red onion. *Coffea* from coffee bean is one of the many remedies for insomnia. *Apis*, a great remedy for bee stings, is made from the honeybee. Other remedies are made from materials as dissimilar as iron, anemones, and the venom of the bushmaster snake. When toxic substances are the origin of a remedy, they are present in such dilute amounts that the remedies are still classified as GRAS (generally recognized as safe) by the FDA.

The homeopathic remedies that are available over the counter at health food stores or pharmacies, or by mail order are generally low potency. They cause no side effects or drug interactions and are only dangerous if used instead of a conventional medical intervention that is clearly needed. Parents interested in using homeopathic remedies to care for their kids' minor illnesses can otherwise experiment with them without doing harm. In addition, it's important to know that—unlike herbal remedies—homeopathic remedies have been regulated tightly by the federal government, just like pharmaceutical agents, for over seventy years.

Just be sure to *contact your child's doctor* at the first sign of something more serious brewing.

If you are interested in using homeopathic remedies for family self-care, do a little research first by reading a few books or taking a class or a mail-order course. (See Resources.) A good reference book can help you decide which remedies are called for in which situations. In choosing a single remedy, consider the person who has the illness—and not just the illness. Ask your child questions like:

- What were you doing before this started?
- How do you feel about this illness? Are you worried or frightened?
- How does your whole body feel? Are you hungry, thirsty, or sleepy?
- What are your specific symptoms?
- Do you feel better in warm places or cool ones?
- Do you feel better sitting up or lying down, on your left side or your right?
- Are there any foods you're craving or foods that disgust you right now?

Look for the remedy that covers the widest number of symptoms. Once you have chosen a remedy, give your child a dose per the package instructions. Stop giving the remedy as soon as symptoms begin to abate and your child is on the path to healing. If symptoms do not improve after three doses properly spaced, rethink your choice of remedy and try again. *Call your pediatrician* if symptoms persist for more than three days or worsen. Keep track of what works for each of your kids, so you know what to try first the next time the same symptoms occur.

TIP: Don't be so free with the use of your homeopathic medicine kit (or any therapy, for that matter) that your children develop the idea that every physical and emotional condition requires some form of medication. Physical and emotional balance is a dynamic process, and we generally have the ability to right most problems ourselves, without the help of outside forces.

A HOMEOPATHIC FIRST AID KIT

Ready-made kits are available, but if you want to put one together for your family, here are a few common remedies that could come in handy when treating children. Use as directed on the label:

Anas barbariae—influenza (often sold as Oscillococcinum)

Chamomilla—teething, insomnia, colic

Arnica—bruises and sports injuries

Allium cepa—colds, hay fever

Euphrasia—irritated eyes, conjunctivitis, hay fever

Apis—bee stings, burns, hives

Hypericum—slamming finger in car door, toothache, sinus pain

Gelsemium—summer colds, fever, headache

Rhus toxicodendron—sprains, strains, and tendonitis when worse after rest

Ruta graveolens—sprains, strains, and tendonitis when better with rest

Aconite—sudden acute inflammation when patient is frightened or anxious

Nux vomica—indigestion, nausea, stomachache

Pulsatilla—ear infections and upper respiratory infections

The individual or combination remedies available to laypeople are most commonly little sugar or lactose pellets or tablets, or liquid formulas. The letters X or C on the label of a homeopathic remedy indicate its strength. Most homeopathic remedies for self-care are 6X, 12X, or 30C.

Oral remedies are taken sublingually (under the tongue). To take pellets or tablets, tap the suggested dosage into the cap of the bottle, then pour the remedy out of the cap into the child's mouth. Have the child keep the pellets or tablets under her tongue until they dissolve. Liquids are dropped from a dropper or the disposable container into the mouth under the tongue. There are also topical homeopathic products such as gels and creams for such conditions as diaper rash, itching, bruising, and muscular soreness.

If you don't want to deal with the process of choosing a single remedy, buy a combination remedy, which includes two or more remedies commonly used to treat the condition. Combined treatment is not as well targeted as a single remedy, however, and it will not work at all if the correct single remedy for your child is not one of the ones included in the formula. That's one reason we lean more toward the single-remedy than the combination approach.

Once again, we suggest that parents give their children over-the-counter homeopathic remedies only for first aid (either as treatment or as a holding action while on the way to the doctor or emergency department) or for minor self-limiting illnesses—the same sorts of situations where you might otherwise turn to herbal remedies or over-the-counter medications.

Energy Medicine

The term *energy medicine* may not be familiar to you. It's a relatively new field of research, though not of practice, as cultural traditions of "energy" healing go back thousands of years. Initially we were both extremely skeptical about the concept, but we have become more open to the idea now that we have watched energy healers at work, experienced the therapy ourselves, and heard good reports from our patients.

Simply put, energy medicine is based on the concept that we are energetic beings in an energetic universe—that we continuously interact with the life energy of the universe and produce subtle energy ourselves through our thoughts and actions—and that this life energy can be sensed and manipulated for health and wellness.

The concept of human energy fields may seem really weird, but we already have the language to talk about it. For instance, we talk of a person as having "personal magnetism," or a place as having "bad vibes." We talk about two people being "in sync," or "on the same wave length." We refer to people or events that really "drain our energy." We have felt the "click" of instant rapport with a new acquaintance or sensed when someone was watching us. We have had our own mood influenced by the anger, anxiety, or grief of others.

As doctors, we know the effect that a health care worker's "energy" can have on a patient. A doctor who comes into her office hurried and distracted will not have the same therapeutic effect as a physician who greets her patient with a smile and a warm handshake. We also have seen how often the "negative" or "positive" energy of a parent (or their anxiety) affects our office interaction with the family, and even the course of the child's illness.

But what does all this talk of energy have to do with medicine? There are entire medical philosophies, like TCM, that are grounded in the idea that good health depends on an unimpeded flow of vital energy through the body. Practitioners of energy therapies such as Jin Shin Jyutsu and Reiki take a somewhat different perspective, believing that they can channel "universal energy" from the outside to stimulate a patient's healing potential. Spiritual healing practices such as prayer, ritual, and the laying on of hands seem to us to have an energetic component too, although it is a Higher Power rather than a nonspecific universal energy that is being accessed.

We're on shaky ground scientifically here, because we are talking about energies that often can't yet be measured by scientific instruments. We have no way to directly measure the power of a prayer or the blockage of qi. We can look only at the results of these therapies, see that something otherwise inexplicable has happened, and theorize about the cause.

There are those who consider the concept of energy medicine sheer poppycock. Yet some of the most important tools of Western diagnostic medicine rely on the fact that the unseen energy produced by the human body can be perceived and measured by sensitive machines. Electrocardiography (EKG), electroencephalography (EEG), and electromyography (EMG) record the electrical energy emitted by the heart, brain, and muscles, respectively. Thermal diagnostics measure heat production, and Doppler scanners pick up sound waves. Biofeedback programs record any of several kinds of body energy.

Conventional medicine also accepts the idea that energy can heal. We use ultrasound waves to reduce inflammation, laser light waves to repair or surgically remove tissue, electricity to speed bone healing or restart a stopped heart, vibration to improve bone density, heat to ease pain, and radiation to cure cancer. By our use of these therapies we acknowledge the ability of certain forms of energy to make changes at the cellular level.

The Basics of Energy Medicine

Research in the field of energy medicine is still scanty, but these are the basic assumptions:

- There is a life force or energy in the universe that permeates everything and everyone.
- Illness, emotion, or physical problems can interrupt the free flow of that force, and vice versa.
- Our bodies produce subtle forms of energy that can travel beyond the body.
- Exposure to even low levels of energy (electrical, magnetic, sound, light, radioactivity) can affect body processes.
- People can intentionally transfer or conduct energy to others with or without touching them.
- One person's energy can be perceived, assessed, and influenced positively by another.
- The transfer or conduction of healing energy requires the presence of good intentions.

Finding a Practitioner

We have seen promising evidence for some forms of energy medicine, and others are simply too wacky for us to even consider. We think it's fine to experiment with energy medicine as long as it is only used for complementary care and not as a replacement for conventional treatment, and as long as it doesn't drain your pocketbook. Most of our patients report benefit from these therapies, even though it may come from nothing more than the opportunity to share time with a compassionate practitioner who is interested in their well-being. Energy therapies properly done appear to help people cope with difficult times, ease stress, lessen pain and anxiety, and speed healing. While some researchers feel that distant, or energy, healing reflects a strong placebo effect, we believe that something more is involved.

Typically a practitioner of energy medicine will begin by "centering" or "grounding" herself to focus her concentration, establish her intention, and either open herself to an energy source (such as the universe, or a Higher Power) or strengthen her own compassionate sensitivities. She will then usually assess the energetic field of her patient, by touch or not, and evaluate the situation. She will attempt to "collect" energy, and then—acting as a passive conduit—transmit or manipulate energy to strengthen or balance the patient. The patient, who is clothed, may feel nothing at all during this treatment, or may feel tingling, warmth, or a sense of relaxation and well-being.

Ask your child's doctor or people you trust for referrals, however, as this is definitely territory where charlatans roam. There are practitioners with excellent training and credentials who have a strong desire to heal, there are "practitioners" who set up shop with little training but a strong desire to make a buck, and there are "practitioners" with good intentions but no skills or a reliance on bizarre machines. In controversial areas such as this, clearly the buyer must beware. As attitude and intention are important to energy healing, look for a practitioner who shares your values and with whom you feel a sympathetic "click." If you cannot find one, consider learning some of these techniques yourself through books, classes, or videos.

Forms of Energy Healing

We have already discussed Chinese, osteopathic, homeopathic, and chiropractic medicine, which all include aspects of energy medicine. Now we'll briefly introduce you to three intriguing forms of energy healing with which you may not be familiar and talk about one very familiar method of healing, prayer. We consider some of these therapies to be "secular," because their practitioners believe they tap into a universal energy to help unblock or strengthen a person's own internal flow of energy (chi), or open or balance energy centers known as "chakras." Others are more spiritual, in that the energy transmitted is assumed to come from a Higher

Power. Give a wide berth to anyone who claims to be the source of healing energy, rather than a conduit. (See Resources for further information about these therapies.)

Therapeutic Touch

A nurse and a spiritual healer were inspired by both the Judeo-Christian practice of laying on hands and the ancient Hindu practice of manipulating body energy to create this secular form of healing. The basic idea of *Therapeutic Touch* (TT) is that interruptions in the free flow of universal energy through the body can be perceived and modified by trained professionals and lay people. Therapeutic Touch and a related form of energy healing called *Healing Touch* are practiced by nurses the world over and can be used by parents and children for self-care as well.

A session of TT lasts about twenty minutes, less for children. After centering herself and becoming attuned to a patient's energy fields, the TT practitioner will move her hands over and around the patient's body about two to four inches from the skin, feeling for places that are colder (energy deficient) or thicker (energy congested). She will then employ techniques to "unruffle" or "smooth" the energy field, sending intentional energy to correct imbalances and assist or otherwise support healing.

Reiki

Based on ancient Tibetan practices, this form of healing was developed about a century ago by a Japanese minister and educator. Reiki (pronounced *ray-kee*) is based on the idea that practitioners can channel the energy of the universal life force for healing through the gentle use of their hands, either by touch or from a distance. Practitioners of Reiki are either lay people or medical professionals who have taken brief training courses that prepare them to work on their own energy, treat others, or train others. (The training required to call oneself a "Reiki Master" is in no way analogous to a master's degree.)

A Reiki treatment will typically take sixty to ninety minutes. The practitioner will usually begin at the patient's head and assess the energy at each of the chakras, transmitting energy when appropriate for health, with the goal of balancing and toning the system. One or two sessions should be enough for relaxation, general tune-ups, or for acute conditions; chronic problems may take longer.

Jin Shin Jyutsu

Like the other forms of energy medicine we're discussing, Jin Shin Jyutsu claims only to help balance "life energy." Practitioners neither diagnose nor treat illness per se. Providers evaluate twelve pulses in the wrist to determine which of a person's twenty-six "safety energy locks" need to be opened or adjusted by a series of gentle hand placements at trouble spots. A typical Jin Shin Jyutsu session will last about an hour. Certain simple positions can be learned and used by anyone—even children—as self-help.

Prayer

In all the healing therapies covered in this chapter something invisible, immeasurable, and powerful appears to be at work. Each talks of accessing an energy or power outside ourselves, be it the Creator, some vital force, or universal life energy.

The earliest physicians were both healers and spiritual leaders. With the advent of scientific medicine, doctors set aside their traditional spiritual roles so completely that issues of spirituality are now seldom brought up in conversations between doctors and patients. We regret this split, because it robs a doctor of an important healing tool.

As integrative physicians we believe strongly that spirit plays a role both in sickness and in healing and can be appropriately discussed in nearly any healing encounter provided it is the patient or family member who introduces the subject. Spirituality, in any of its forms, can help parents and children find comfort in a trying situation, increase their sense of connection to others and the world around them, and provide them with hope, meaning, and even a greater appreciation for life's magic. A physician who honors and enlists a patient's own unique spiritual practice can augment even conventional medical treatment.

Fortunately, in the past few years there's been a sea change in the attitude of the medical establishment toward spirituality, due to an increasing number of scientific studies on the topic and an increased desire on the part of patients to bring their spiritual tools into their health care. Today more than fifty medical schools offer courses in spirituality and medicine. Researchers at Duke, Harvard, and other top universities have linked religious faith or spirituality to greater optimism, greater coping skills, greater resilience in the face of stress, greater perceived social support, lower levels of anxiety, and a longer, healthier life. We think there may be other factors at work here as well (religious people may have a better sense of connection to the community or may just take better care of themselves), but we do believe that it is both important and healthy for children to be taught a sense of spiritual (although not necessarily religious) connection to others and to the universe, and to be given spiritual tools. We feel that personal or communal prayer can be an important complement to medical therapy but not a substitute for it.

Although a majority of American adults say a doctor should address a patient's spiritual needs, no patient wants to feel pressure to adhere to the doctor's own beliefs. But we think it is often appropriate and even helpful to ask a patient and his parents such questions as: When things are difficult, where do you turn for comfort? What gives you strength? Is your spiritual life important to you? Do you have a regular spiritual or religious practice? How would you like me as your doctor to address these issues in your health care? The goal with these questions is to identify the spiritual tools at a patient's command so they can be mobilized for her recovery. You may think these questions are too deep for children, but in our experience, kids have spiritual values and resources, too.

THE DIFFERENCE BETWEEN HEALING AND CURING

We want to make clear the distinction between "healing" and "curing." A *cure* gets rid of all physical signs of an illness. *Healing*, on the other hand, goes beyond the physical to encompass the emotional, psychological, and spiritual aspects of an illness as well. A disease does not have to disappear for a person to feel healed. We consider that healing has occurred if a patient has come to feel whole and blessed and alive, even if the disease still exists in the body. We have both cared for exceptional patients who taught us that dying and healing are not in fact incompatible, experiences that were life changing for us.

How can spirituality be used for healing? We believe that most illnesses—physical, emotional, and psychological—have a spiritual component. Such spiritual conflicts as issues of trust, faith, guilt, forgiveness, and reconciliation can express themselves as physical or psychological disease. In addition, many times a disease can cause a spiritual crisis. But most important, spiritual rituals and tools can help with healing.

People of faith have different spiritual tools at their command. These tools—loosely described as personal prayer or meditation, prayer by others (intercessory prayer), ritual, or contact with a holy book, person, or place—can be exceptionally powerful. Prayer and meditation are especially effective therapy for any condition that is made worse or caused by stress, such as pain, infertility, insomnia, anxiety, and depression. Best of all, prayer is a two-way street, offering benefits both to the person praying and the person prayed for. We both include our patients in our private prayers, and will pray with families during a visit if asked.

We don't know if it will ever be scientifically proven that prayer speeds healing, but we know it gives us something positive to do when we feel powerless, and it allows an outlet for our feelings of love and compassion for others. And who's to say that a mother praying for her son's recovery is not transmitting healing energy that will make a difference in the course of his illness?

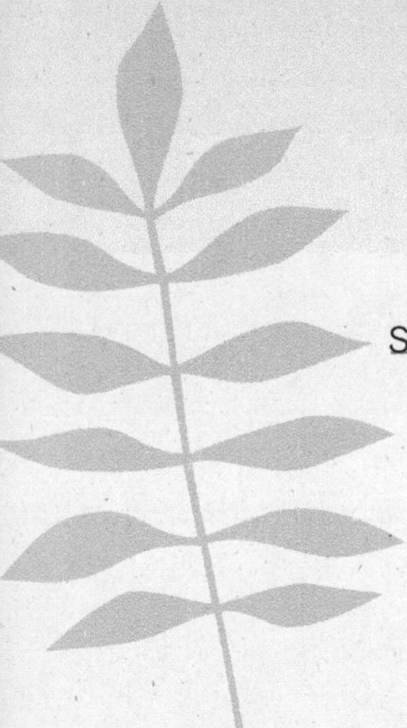

SECTION III

conditions

CHAPTER 14

Colds, Flu, and Other Respiratory Illnesses

No wonder we associate runny noses with little kids! The average young child gets six to ten colds a year, tapering off to two to four a year as he or she nears adulthood. Children get more colds and other respiratory illnesses than we do because their developing immune systems haven't yet learned to recognize cold viruses and organize an effective defense against them. By the time your children are old enough to vote, you'll probably have dealt with at least a hundred runny noses, hacking coughs, and feverish flus.

Respiratory illnesses affect the nose, mouth, sinuses, windpipe (trachea), the two airways that lead to the lobes of the lungs (bronchi), the smaller airways within the lungs (bronchioles), and/or the air-filled sacs (alveoli) that give the lung its spongy appearance. In this chapter we briefly discuss common conditions of the upper respiratory tract (colds, croup, sinusitis) and the lower respiratory tract (bronchitis, bronchiolitis, and pneumonia), as well as one total-body flattener (influenza).

The most important thing to remember is that respiratory infections are usually caused by viruses. This means that antibiotics are useless at curing colds, flu, and most cases of bronchitis. In fact, they can actually makes things worse by upsetting the normal healthy balance among the many bacteria that live within our bodies.

Even healthy children will get at least a few mild respiratory illnesses and suffer symptoms that make both child and parent very unhappy. You should do what you can to ease your child's symptoms, but know that, given time, these mild, self-limiting infections will resolve on their own in an otherwise healthy child. Our treatment advice is therefore simple: Rest and keep the body hydrated. Encourage your child to sleep as much as possible to allow the immune system time and energy to battle the virus. Give moderate amounts of clear fluids—water, broth, juice, even juice pops—to flush the body of toxins and provide the moisture the tissues lining the respiratory tract need to repel viruses effectively.

While the common respiratory illnesses usually clear up on their own with a little time, parents should still stay alert for any worsening of symptoms, as complications can occur or what seems at first like a cold may actually be something else altogether.

Call your child's physician if symptoms last longer than a week, if fever returns after the initial fever has wound down, if your child cannot keep fluids down or has pain in the face or teeth. *Go to the emergency department or call 911* if a child complains of chest pains, has difficulty breathing or is breathing very rapidly, has a bluish cast to his or her skin (cyanosis), or is not behaving normally.

With that general introduction, let's move on to specifics about symptoms, prevention, and integrative treatment of the more common forms of respiratory illness.

more on . . .

COLDS AND STRESS

Although we are all exposed to the viruses that cause colds and other respiratory illnesses, those who are under stress or run-down are far more likely to actually get them. That's why it's so important to eat well and get enough sleep during the late fall and winter months we call the cold and flu season. That's the time of year you'll want to be especially careful to keep up the immune-boosting strategies we discussed in chapter 2.

Upper Respiratory Infections

The Common Cold

Almost all of the common respiratory infections seem to start out as a cold, which is formally defined as a viral infection of the mucous membranes of the nose, sinuses, throat, and upper airway. Someone with a cold may have a runny nose, tearing eyes, scratchy throat, cough, congestion, sneezing, poor appetite, or mild fever, and may just feel "icky." A cold in a young child generally lasts about a week but can last significantly longer. Most colds are uncomplicated and resolve completely.

Prevention

It would be nice if we had a vaccine that could prevent the common cold, but that's unlikely, because there are about 200 viruses that can cause one. Colds are very contagious, with viruses being spread through sneezing (they can travel 12 feet!) or hand-to-hand or hand-to-object contact. Very young children get more colds not only because their immune systems are still being educated but also because they don't wash their hands often, tend to wipe their noses with their arms or a sleeve, and have a lot of physical contact with their playmates. The good news is that this exchange of common viruses may help most children build a healthy immune system. The bad news is that they catch half a dozen colds a year.

more on . . .

MUCUS

The mucus (or colloquially, snot) draining from our noses that we associate with a cold is actually a defensive tactic. Early on, when a cold is at its most contagious, the clear and watery mucus is chock full of viruses being flushed out of the body. Later the mucus becomes thicker and whitish or yellowish because it is also full of dead immune cells that have fought the offending virus. Parents often worry that thick, yellowish or greenish mucus signals a bacterial infection in the sinuses, but this is not always the case. We don't worry unless we also see more serious symptoms, such as high fever and facial pain or swelling, which might indicate a bacterial sinus infection.

The best ways to prevent a cold are:

- Wash hands often and well (see chapter 4) with simple liquid soap, especially before meals or snacks. Skip alcohol-based hand gels as they dry out tender skin.
- Teach children to cover their mouths when they sneeze or cough, and then to wash their hands.
- Limit exposure to airborne pollutants like secondhand tobacco smoke.
- Regularly practice effective stress-management techniques (see chapter 10).
- Get plenty of sleep each night.
- Stay social. It's a myth that you should stay indoors and away from people during cold and flu season. Research suggests that being around friends and loved ones may actually help boost our immune systems.

Treatment

We believe that the best treatment for self-limiting illnesses is to get out of the way and let the natural forces of healing do their work. You can sometimes avert or reduce the severity or duration of a cold by taking quick action in its early stages. (Though we have used these remedies with positive results, in some cases solid data is still missing on their safety or efficacy in children, or on the optimal dosage.)

- *Vitamin* C. At the first sign of a cold, feed your child foods high in vitamin C, such as orange juice or citrus fruit, kiwi, strawberries and other berries, melon, bell peppers, and broccoli, to try to shorten its duration. Alternatively, you can give a child a quick-loading dose of vitamin C (100 mg total per day for a toddler or 200 mg a day for an older child) when he first notices a scratchy throat or sniffle.

TIP: The most kid-friendly forms of vitamin C are chewable tablets or "gummies" and powdered vitamin C mixed in water or juice. Make sure kids brush their teeth or rinse out their mouths after taking any chewable to avoid tooth damage by the ascorbic acid.

▶ *Echinacea*. The jury is still out on the effectiveness of the herb echinacea (purple coneflower) in lessening the severity or duration of a cold. There are many questions as to which dose, product, variety, and part of the plant—if any—is optimal, and studies on its efficacy are conflicting, but we are confident enough about its safety and effectiveness to give this remedy to our own children. It seems to work better in some folks than in others, but since there is no effective treatment for the common cold, it's worth seeing if it works for your children. We recommend 6 to 8 drops of a standardized liquid extract or tincture of echinacea in water or juice two to five times a day for kids aged two to six. The dose is 8 to 15 drops at a time for kids aged seven to twelve. Start at the first sign of symptoms and continue for no more than seven days. There is no evidence that it is useful to take for the full cold season as a general preventive. (Children with autoimmune disorders or known allergies to plants in the ragweed family should not take echinacea until studies disprove theoretical concerns about their using the herb.)

▶ *Garlic*. Put lots of this excellent antimicrobial fresh in foods, or give your kids ½ teaspoon of a liquid garlic extract such as Kyolic (for kids one to five, older kids can take a full teaspoon) in grape juice twice a day.

▶ *Asian herbal extracts*. Dr. D sometimes uses a special liquid extract of the Japanese medicinal mushroom maitake (called maitake d-fraction) to help abort a cold. He puts 5 drops in a teaspoon of chocolate syrup (helps make the medicine go down) three times a day for children one to five years old (10 drops for children six and over). Dr. Russ sometimes suggests use of North American ginseng (*Panax quinquefolius*) to prevent colds in older children. Another herb used against the common cold in Asia is *Andrographis paniculata*, sometimes combined with North American ginseng.

TIP: Is it a cold or an allergy? Both can cause sneezing, stuffy nose, scratchy throat, and reddened eyes. Colds peak in the late fall and winter and last about a week. Allergies last longer and can occur anytime, although often at the same time each year (grass or pollen allergies). Allergies can also leave you more susceptible to colds. Mild fever or body aches typically signal a cold; itchy eyes or itchy skin point to allergy. (For more on allergic rhinitis, see chapter 20.)

Congestion

We don't recommend antihistamines or other over-the-counter medicines for congestion, even for children over the age of six (for whom the FDA has approved their use). Although decongestants generally decrease swelling in the nasal cavities and make breathing a little easier, we believe they sidetrack the natural healing process. In addition, they have many potential side effects, including irritability, increased blood pressure, and rapid heart rate. These drugs offer four to six hours of relief at most, and can cause increased mucus production and congestion (the "rebound" effect) if used for more than five days. We give decongestants (primarily pseudoephedrine) only when a child over six has severe discomfort.

We recommend natural measures to reduce the congestion of a cold:

- Use nasal aspirators (inexpensive little rubber bulbs) to suction excess mucus from the nose of a baby with a cold. Young children can also use the bulb together with a store-bought or homemade saline solution to clean out the nasal passages. Just mix ¼ teaspoon table salt in a cup of warm water and use five or six times a day to loosen thickened nasal secretions and allow for freer breathing. This is especially useful with nursing babies who cannot eat if they cannot breathe. (For older children we recommend the neti pots described below.)

- Older children should be taught the fine art of gently blowing one's nose so as not to send germ-laden mucus up into the ears or sinuses. If nose blowing leads to a raw nose, use petroleum jelly, aloe gel, calendula cream, or other salve.

- Get plenty of rest.

▶ Drink lots of liquids. Don't forget chicken soup—studies suggest that your grandmother's favorite remedy really does improve cold symptoms.

▶ Use steam to soothe and moisturize nasal passages and open sinuses. A cool-mist vaporizer can moisturize the air in your child's bedroom; be sure to clean well after use so molds do not grow in it. Or you can run a very hot shower and let your child sit in the bathroom and breathe in the steam.

▶ Consider experimenting with a homeopathic remedy, choosing one that suits your child's symptoms.

TIP: Older children may benefit from irrigating their nose and sinuses using a neti pot (available in many health food stores) and some homemade saline solution (see above). Have your child stand over the sink, turn her head to one side while compressing the lower nostril, and pour the liquid from the neti pot into the upper nostril as she gives a short snort inward. Then have her release the lower nostril and let all the fluid (and associated gunk) drain out. Repeat on the other side. It sounds gross, but it really isn't uncomfortable and can be very effective at clearing out nasal passages and sinuses.

Cough

Like a runny nose, a cough is a defensive mechanism. It clears the throat and airways of obstructions and foreign matter to allow better breathing. Much of the cold-related coughing in children is in response to the scratchy, irritable sensation caused by mucus dripping down the back of throat. The cough caused by postnasal drip tends to flare up when the child is lying flat, causing nighttime coughing and sleeplessness for child and parent alike.

We don't generally advise trying to suppress the coughs that accompany colds. The cough is helping rid the body of irritants. Furthermore, over-the-counter cough medicines don't cure a cough, they just stifle it (suppressants) or cause it to be more "productive" (expectorants). These medicines have significant side effects and are not always effective for children. While they are safe in pediatric doses, it is easy to take an overdose. We occasionally prescribe cough suppressants, but only in situations where a child older than five is just not getting any sleep because of a cough.

We rarely recommend expectorants except for the occasional case where a child with bronchitis needs help expelling mucus from his lungs. The active ingredient of many expectorants is guaifenesin. Although the drug does thin mucus, in our experience it often causes more profuse postnasal drip and increased coughing in kids.

Here's a more natural approach to reducing discomfort associated with cough:

- ▶ Encourage your child to blow his or her nose frequently (and gently) to avoid postnasal drip.
- ▶ Rest and drink lots of liquids. Warm fluids like broths, teas, and heated juices may be best because they enhance blood flow, soothe the throat, and replace liquids lost in the course of illness.
- ▶ A cool-mist vaporizer in your child's room can ease a cough, as can elevating the head of your child's bed or crib (or tucking a folded blanket or pillow under the head end of the crib mattress).
- ▶ Lozenges can ease the throat tickle that triggers a cough. In addition to the familiar cough drops of all sorts, we also like the cherry-flavored lozenges made of slippery elm, an herb that soothes the mucous membranes.
- ▶ Liquid extract of slippery elm is a useful herbal treatment for coughs. Give children aged two to four a ½ teaspoon twice a day, and older kids 1 teaspoon twice a day until the throat feels better. You can also mix 1 teaspoon of slippery elm powder with 1 tablespoon of sugar, a sprinkle of cinnamon, and 2 cups of boiling water for a soothing drink that can be sipped (once cooled) throughout the day. Mullein tea is another traditional herbal remedy for coughs.
- ▶ A teaspoonful of honey at bedtime can help quell a cough and help your child get some sleep. Do not give honey to children under one year of age (to avoid a deadly disease caused botulism).

A persistent cough may be a sign of something more than a cold, such as gastroesophageal reflux (GERD), foreign body aspiration, or reactive airway disease. *Call your child's physician* for any cough in an infant under three months, or for a cough in an older child that causes wheezing or other breathing problems, comes with high fever, or lasts longer than two weeks.

Fever

Sometimes a cold is accompanied by a fever. The fever is not itself an illness, but a natural defensive reaction against infection. Many parents are frightened by fever and start giving antifever medications as soon as a child's temperature goes above 98.6° F. They forget that some children normally run a little hotter or cooler than 98.6° F (which is just an average) and that body temperature will normally be a little higher in the evening than in the morning. Besides, low-grade fever by itself is rarely harmful.

Not all fevers need to be treated. We don't normally treat children over a year old with any medications for low-grade fever unless the child is very uncomfortable or looks sick, although clearly you should consult a doctor if your child's fever is prolonged or very high. We suggest a dose of children's acetaminophen or ibuprofen appropriate for the child's weight. (Never give aspirin to a child who might have a viral illness because of the risk of a liver-damaging disease called Reyes Syndrome.) Be sure to use the dropper or measuring cap that came with the medicine, or a measuring spoon (not a teaspoon from your silverware drawer), and give the correct dose for the form (drops, elixir, or chewable). Continue giving acetaminophen or ibuprofen every four to six hours as directed until your child starts to feel better or the fever goes down. The purpose of the acetaminophen is purely to make your child more comfortable, so there's no reason to wake up a sleeping child for another dose.

When Should Parents Worry about a Fever?

It is very common for a child to spike a fever of 103 to 105° F for a fairly benign virus. When parents call Dr. D about feverish children, he always asks whether the child can still be made to smile when the fever abates. If so, he feels reasonably certain that the fever is not being caused by a serious bacterial infection. Fevers rarely go high enough to cause lasting harm except in situations where there is also interference with a child's heating and cooling mechanisms, such as when a feverish child is wrapped in too many blankets or a child is left in a closed car on a hot day.

For the mild fever that may accompany colds, rest and liquids are especially important; juice popsicles feel especially good. Sponge a very hot child with a washcloth dipped in lukewarm water and wrung out—never use cold water or alcohol, as the sudden temperature change can be a shock to your child's system and even cause a seizure.

Call your child's physician immediately for a child under three months of age who has a fever of 100.6° F (rectal) or more, a child three to six months old who has a fever over 101° F (rectal), or an older child who has had a fever over 103° F (oral) for more than a day or a bad headache associated with the fever. Call if your child has suffered a seizure from the fever and has a history of same, or if a feverish child shows a rash.

Call 911 or go to the emergency department if a child suffers the seizure that can sometimes occur as a result of a rapidly rising fever, has never had this before, and you cannot contact your physician, or if a feverish child has trouble breathing, turns blue, is in pain, or delirious.

Sinus Pain

The sinus cavities are air-filled pockets within the bony structure of the skull located above the eyes, behind the cheeks and to the sides of the nasal passages. The sinuses make mucus, which is then swept into the nose by tiny hairs called cilia that line the respiratory passages. A child's cold will often be accompanied by at least mild pain in the forehead or face from an excess of mucus in the sinuses or an obstruction in the flow of mucus. To relieve cold-related sinus pain, you can:

- Place warm washcloths on the face over the sinuses.

- Give children's acetaminophen or ibuprofen at dosages indicated on package labels to relieve more severe sinus pain.

▶ Massage the chest of a child over the age of three with an over-the-counter decongestant herbal aromatic rub or one made by mixing a drop of essential oil of eucalyptus in an ounce of a vegetable or nut oil such as olive or almond oil. (Do not apply essential oils undiluted to a child's skin.) Don't use the rub on the face, where it can get into the mucous membranes, which can be dangerous. If you prefer, you can rub a drop of eucalyptus oil on your child's blanket at bedtime to relieve congestion.

▶ Give an over-the-counter decongestant such as pseudoephedrine for up to five days. This is perhaps the only instance when we do recommend decongestants. We may also prescribe nonsedating antihistamines if symptoms persist for kids over the age of six.

▶ Try acupuncture. Dr. Russ has seen some astonishing results in the treatment of acute sinusitis, with clogged sinuses starting to drain freely during a treatment.

▶ Cranial osteopathy (described in chapter 11) provides excellent relief of symptoms for chronic sinusitis and may prevent recurrence.

▶ Use a neti pot or other method of irrigation as described on page 215 to clear sinuses.

The sinus problems that accompany a cold can sometimes turn into something more serious because the mucus backed up in the sinuses creates a friendly incubator for bacteria. It can be difficult then for a physician to tell whether or not the problem is bacterial sinusitis, which should be treated with antibiotics. Fortunately, viral sinusitis is 20 to 200 times more likely than bacterial sinusitis in children. Some doctors recommend an X-ray, CT scan, or MRI to determine the presence of more severe bacterial sinusitis, but interpretation of the images is very difficult because young children have poorly developed sinus cavities and may show abnormally fluid-filled sinuses even with routine colds or allergies.

Call your child's physician if your child has facial or dental pain or a fever that returns after initial cold symptoms have subsided. In cases such as these, we often do prescribe antibiotics, as these are symptoms that may be associated with a bacterial sinus infection. We start with the simplest form of antibiotic (amoxicillin) and advance to stronger, broad-spectrum antibiotics only if no improvement is noted in the first three to five days. Be sure that any child on antibiotics takes the full course, even if symptoms disappear before the prescription is finished. Antibiotics for sinusitis need to be taken longer than usual, preferably two to three weeks. We usually recommend that these patients eat lots of yogurt (fresh or frozen) with live cultures, or take a probiotic supplement with lactobacilli or bifidobacteria, to re-establish the beneficial intestinal bacteria ("good bugs") killed by the medication.

Croup

Croup is a viral illness that usually starts with coldlike symptoms before progressing to swelling and inflammation of the vocal cords and windpipe. It can also come on without warning, with its distinctive cough the first sign. Croup occurs most often in the cold-and-flu days of winter, and is always worse at night. The most obvious symptom of croup is the notorious barking cough and restricted breathing that terrify both kids and parents at 2 A.M. The child may have significant hoarseness (laryngitis) and/or a moderate fever as well.

Although it is frightening to hear your little munchkin suddenly sound like a walrus, there are a number of things you can do to relieve croup symptoms. Among them:

- *Steam*. Turn the shower on to full hot, close the bathroom door, and sit outside the shower with your little barking child in the steam-filled room until his cough eases. Turn the cool-mist humidifier on in his room for the rest of the night.

- *Cold*. Cold can break up a coughing spasm. If it's cold out, wrap your child up and carry her around outside for ten or fifteen minutes.

- *Relaxation techniques*. Slow breathing or an imagery exercise can reduce your child's anxiety and slow his respiratory rate. Anxiety aggravates respiratory distress, so keeping your child (and yourself) calm is critical to relieving symptoms of croup.

Generally, croup is another viral self-limiting illness that will resolve in a few days and can be treated at home with the guidance of a pediatrician. The frightening barking cough is usually followed by several days of a wet, looser, and less restrictive cough. Some kids have a tendency toward croup, but they usually outgrow it by age six.

Call your child's physician or *go to the emergency room* if your child is having severe difficulty with breathing that does not ease with steam or cold air. Warning signs include a high-pitched sound when breathing in (stridor), skin between the ribs being drawn in with each inhalation, or agitated behavior or confusion. Advanced cases of croup will require steroid treatment; occasionally a child is admitted to the hospital for further monitoring.

Lower Respiratory Infections

Bronchitis

The term *bronchitis* refers to swelling or inflammation of the bronchi, the major airways in the lungs through which oxygen flows in and carbon dioxide flows out. Most cases of bronchitis are actually colds with predominant bronchial symptoms such as chest congestion, chest discomfort, cough, and, often, wheezing. Because colds and bronchitis so frequently overlap, we are careful not to overtreat any child who appears reasonably comfortable or is not in respiratory distress. We advise parents to help relieve symptoms (see our approach to colds and coughs above), and keep an eye on the child to make sure the situation does not worsen.

TIP: Although frightening to parents, wheezing is not necessarily serious, as air is still flowing in and out of the child's lungs. It is actually more serious when a wheezing child stops wheezing but still has difficulty breathing, as it means that the airways are now so restricted that there is not enough air going through them to even cause a wheeze.

We don't usually treat bronchitis any differently than a cold, recommending rest and plenty of liquids. Short-term use of some herbal remedies, like African geranium (*Pelargonium sidoides*), echinacea, or North American ginseng, may be of benefit. If a child's wheezing or distress is significant, we may prescribe a bronchodilating agent, such as albuterol, to ease breathing; these medications come as nebulizers, metered-dose inhalers, or in liquid form.

We do not hand out prescriptions for antibiotics for most children with bronchitis, as it is generally a self-limiting viral illness that does not respond to antibiotics. There are exceptions, however. For instance, children with chronic lung diseases, such as cystic fibrosis, do generally require an antibiotic for bronchial symptoms due to underlying lung damage and mucus stagnation, which could lead to bacterial overgrowth. And occasionally a bacterium will set up shop in the bronchi of an otherwise healthy child. We decide whether or not to prescribe antibiotics based on a child's history, current symptoms, physical exam, and a parent's ability to monitor the condition closely and insure proper follow-up.

Bronchiolitis

Bronchiolitis is an inflammation of the smaller airways (bronchioles) deeper in the lungs, which can be caused by a number of viruses, among them *respiratory syncytial virus* (RSV). RSV is a common cause of many upper and lower respiratory infections, including colds and pneumonia. In older kids and adults, RSV is just a nuisance, but in very young children bronchiolitis caused by RSV can progress to a life-threatening illness. It is a significant cause of hospitalizations of children under a year old in the winter and early spring, especially those infants considered high risk due to prematurity or cardiac problems. Such children may require treatment with medications only available at a hospital and should be considered for a vaccine called Synagis that can prevent RSV for the season.

Call your child's physician or *go to the emergency department* for a high-risk infant who has difficulty breathing, turns blue, or has coughing, severe congestion, vomiting, fussiness, or an inability to eat or drink. Children with bronchiolitis may look as if they are having an acute asthma attack; the spaces between their ribs go in and out when they breathe. They need conventional Western medical treatment.

Pertussis (Whooping Cough)

Whooping cough is a preventable bacterial infection that affects the same portion of the airway as bronchiolitis. It too may start with coldlike symptoms, but the hallmark of whooping cough is the "whoop" a child makes when gasping for air after one of the frequent, long-lasting repetitive coughing spells that characterize this disease. The "staccato" coughing (five to ten coughs, one right after another) makes it so hard to take a breath that the child may turn blue from lack of oxygen. Whooping cough is caused not by cold or flu viruses, but by a bacterium (*Bordetella pertussis*). Thanks to vaccination, this potentially life-threatening infection is much less common but still cause for concern in cities or in areas where there are clusters of children unvaccinated for religious or philosophical reasons, inadequately vaccinated immigrants, or adults whose immunity is waning. Anyone over eleven (including adults) should get a booster shot.

Call your child's physician right away if you suspect your child has pertussis based on the symptoms described above. If distress is present, he may ask you to take your child to the emergency department of your local hospital.

Pneumonia

Pneumonia is the result of infected fluids accumulating in the air sacs, or alveoli, at the ends of the airways. In most cases, this infection is accompanied by cough, progressive weakness, rapid breathing, inactivity, poor food and fluid intake, high fever, and sometimes wheezing. Infants may show irritability, lack of appetite, and rapid breathing, but generally their diagnosis comes more from what doctors refer to as "sick-looking-kid" syndrome.

Pneumonia can be caused by a wide variety of organisms, and it is difficult but crucial to determine whether your child is suffering from a bacterial or viral illness when considering treatment possibilities. Viral pneumonias tend to develop more slowly and have less serious symptoms associated with them.

Typically the physician will order a white blood cell count and chest X-ray to help determine whether a child has viral or bacterial pneumonia. While antibiotics are not of use for viral pneumonias, bacterial pneumonia (while less common) is quite aggressive in children and should be treated with appropriate oral antibiotics for mild and moderate cases and a shot or intravenous antibiotics for severe cases. Again, probiotic use during antibiotic treatment may be useful in preventing gastrointestinal side effects.

A few remedies that might be useful for a child with viral pneumonia or as complementary therapy for a child being treated for bacterial pneumonia:

- Rest and lots of fluids
- Use of an herbal tonic, such as echinacea, garlic, or maitake (see chapter 12)
- Breath work to exercise the lungs
- Mind/body exercises, especially hypnosis or guided imagery, to hasten the healing process

Influenza

We don't need to tell you what flu is. Once you've had it, you'll recognize it again. By definition, influenza is a viral illness that comes on suddenly and more severely than a cold and typically lasts a week to ten days. Symptoms include fever, aches, chills, cough, runny nose, sore throat, headache, nausea or vomiting, and a lack of energy or appetite. Most people with flu feel like they've been hit by a truck and just want to stay in bed.

Prevention

The best way to protect your children from flu is for everyone in the family to wash their hands frequently during flu season—from November to April. Influenza is spread easily by person-to-person contact, and hand washing breaks the chain. This is also a good time of year to be especially committed to following the suggestions we gave in chapter 2 for optimizing immune function.

We do recommend annual immunization against influenza for expectant mothers and for children aged six months to five years, using thimerasol-free vaccine. Side effects are generally rare, and the shot offers protection against secondary infection by an antibiotic-resistant bacterium, the most common catastrophic complication of flu. It also protects adults, who mostly get their cases of flu from kids.

Treatment

Most children do not require antiviral prescription drugs for flu. The flu bugs have built up resistance to the older ones (ending in "tidine"), and there are concerns about behavioral changes in those who have taken the newer ones (ending in "amavir"), so we recommend neither. We prefer gentler ways of reducing the severity or duration of the flu. At the first sign of flu, have your child start taking ½ teaspoon of sweet, fruity-tasting elderberry (*Sambucus nigra*) extract two or three times a day for five days. Elderberry extract has compounds that act in unique fashion to help forestall the flu. The homeopathic medicine Oscillococcinum (*Anas barbariae*) is another kid-friendly remedy that can help if started when symptoms first occur; take according to package directions every six hours for eighteen hours.

For symptomatic relief, consider the following:

- *Rest and plenty of fluids*. Keep them comfy in bed so they can nap. See whether your child prefers warm or cool drinks, and keep them coming. Popsicles made of fruit juice are generally welcome, too—there are even new ones that include oral-rehydration therapy. You might try a smoothie as a way to pack more nutrition into those fluids.
- *Children's acetaminophen or ibuprofen for fever, aches, or pain*. Aspirin should be avoided.
- *Massage with a pleasantly scented oil or lotion to relieve aching muscles and joints*. Vanilla, lavender, and chamomile are popular choices.
- *Give maitake and/or garlic as described previously*. Dr. D sometimes uses echinacea as well. A little nibble on some candied ginger, or drinking tea made of minced ginger root and a little honey, can ease nausea in children over a year old.
- *Use a cool-mist humidifier for stuffiness or sore throat.*
- *A cool washcloth feels great on a fevered brow.*
- *Favorite music, videos, or other forms of distraction may help.*

CHAPTER 15

Sore Throat

There are many causes of sore throat, but parents are most concerned about those caused by strep. They know that all their plans for the week will be up in the air while they try to decide if their child needs to see a doctor, which parent will be able to take him, who will stay home with him until he is no longer infectious, and whether or not to have the other kids tested for strep too. Many also know that untreated strep can be dangerous.

A sore throat comes from an infection or inflammation of the tonsils and pharynx, the muscular tube lined by mucous membranes that delivers food and air from the back of the nose and mouth to either the feeding tube (esophagus) that goes to the stomach or the windpipe (trachea) that leads to the lungs. Tucked into each side of the pharynx at the back of the mouth are small lymphoid tissues called the tonsils that help fight infection; the adenoid in the upper throat at the back of the nose serves a similar function. Their job is to respond to offending viral, bacterial, or environmental agents.

Most cases of sore throat are viral in origin and are cleared by our bodies within a few days. Others are caused by environmental insults such as allergens or cigarette smoke, or even by sleeping with the mouth open, which dries out protective mucous membranes. Some are caused by bacteria.

more on . . .

VIRAL OR BACTERIAL?

It can be difficult to tell a viral from a bacterial sore throat just by looking at it and taking a child's history. Either kind of sore throat can cause pain, fever, enlarged lymph nodes, difficulty swallowing, red pharynx with white stuff on the tonsils, and beefy tonsils. Viral sore throat is more likely to come with a cough or runny nose. Bacterial sore throat is more often accompanied by headache, bellyache, nausea, and foul-smelling breath.

Only 15 to 20 percent of sore throats in children are caused by the *Streptococcus* bacterium. While most cases are mild, a strep infection can be life threatening, depending on its location, the virulence of the strain of *Streptococcus*, and the quality of the child's immune response. The majority of cases of strep throat resolve on their own, but we treat all cases of strep throat seriously, because a strep infection can sometimes lead to inflammation or damage to the heart, joints, or skin from rheumatic fever. Treatment with a full course of antibiotics usually prevents these complications and speeds resolution of symptoms.

So the million-dollar question with any sore throat is: Is it caused by a bacterium or a virus? A child can ride out a viral sore throat with just some intervention to relieve pain and other symptoms, but a bacterial sore throat may need to be treated with antibiotics. It's difficult even for a doctor to tell from symptoms alone whether a red or aching throat is caused by a strep infection, so we just regard any sore throat that has lasted for more than 24 hours as suspicious and test for it appropriately. A throat that clears up in less than 48 hours is likely to have had a viral cause, but even a quick resolution is not a guarantee.

Call your child's physician if in addition to a sore throat your child has a fever and swollen glands, a barking cough, a change in his or her voice, or difficulty in swallowing or keeping fluids down.

Go to the emergency department if your child has difficulty breathing or assumes the "sniffing position" (head and neck extended to ease breathing), or appears lethargic or confused.

A test for the presence or absence of Group A beta-hemolytic *Streptococcus*, the strain that causes rheumatic fever and other nasty strep complications, will help determine when an antibiotic is necessary. There are still some doctors who routinely hand out antibiotic prescriptions for acutely sore throats without doing a definitive test, but we are not among them. We do a rapid strep test. If it is positive, we prescribe oral amoxicillin, unless the patient is allergic to penicillin. If the test result is negative, we do a 24-hour throat culture to confirm, as the rapid test is not as accurate as the overnight culture.

When antibiotics are prescribed, it is very important that children take the full course in order to prevent complications or recurrence. We usually recommend a concurrent three-to-four-week course of an over-the-counter probiotic with lactobacilli or bifidobacteria during treatment to protect the normal intestinal flora from being destroyed by the antibiotic.

Here are a few natural remedies to ease a sore throat, once strep has been ruled out or is already being treated:

- Hot or cold liquids can soothe the mucous membranes, increase local blood flow, and keep the body well hydrated. Hot water with honey and lemon (only for children over one year in age) and chicken soup are traditional favorites. Adding chopped fresh garlic to the chicken broth might boost its healing potential. If cold feels better, offer iced noncaffeinated teas, full-strength fruit juices, flavored waters, juice pops, or Pedialyte pops—a frozen form of oral rehydration therapy.
- Food hurt going down? Try slippery foods like rice pudding, Jell-O, or noodles with olive oil and crushed garlic.
- Relieve pain with children's acetaminophen or ibuprofen as directed on the package. Do not use aspirin products.
- Use a cool-mist vaporizer to keep mucous membranes in the throat moist.
- A gargle of either one part hydrogen peroxide to three parts water or ½ teaspoon table salt in a glass of warm water can soothe a child old enough to gargle. Older kids may prefer a low-alcohol mouthwash.
- Immune-boosting herbs can speed healing. You can try echinacea or elderberry extracts (4 to 8 drops of standardized extract in water or juice

two to five times a day for kids two to six, and 8 to 15 drops for kids six to twelve). Garlic may shorten the duration of a sore throat and prevent recurrences, especially for viral illness. Dr. D advises ¼ to ½ teaspoon of liquid garlic extract twice a day for kids eighteen months to three years, or a full teaspoon for kids three to twelve, added to a big glass of fruit or vegetable juice or mixed with a little chocolate- or fruit-flavored syrup to improve the taste. Dr. Russ prefers to crush fresh garlic and add it to salads or to hot foods during the last five minutes of cooking.

▶ Choose a homeopathic remedy that suits your child's symptoms, say, *Apis* for a very red throat that feels better with cold drinks. (See chapter 13.)

▶ Throat lozenges can relieve pain for a short time, and there's a wide variety to try. We prefer the fruit-flavored ones made with the herb slippery elm, which has a long history of soothing sore throats. Older children might find chewing one or two tablets of deglycyrrhizinated licorice (DGL) soothing to an inflamed throat, too.

▶ Massage the outside of the throat with an aromatic herbal rub, perhaps an ounce of vegetable oil with a drop of eucalyptus essential oil in it, but only for kids over three.

▶ Do the Lion, a yoga exercise designed to increase circulation in the throat, as described in chapter 10.

more on . . .

SOME UNEXPECTED CONSEQUENCES OF STREP

If your child develops tics or odd behavior after a strep infection, she may be suffering from a PANDA (pediatric autoimmune neurobehavioral disorder associated with streptococcal infection). A PANDA may express itself as abnormal jerking movements or as obsessive-compulsive behavior. A post-strep blood test can be given, and if it reveals the more prolonged and abnormally high strep-antibody count typical of a PANDA, your child's doctor can prescribe a longer, one-month course of antibiotics to help resolve the symptoms.

CHAPTER 16

Ear Infection

In the days before antibiotic drugs, earaches were treated with various natural remedies. Most healed and went away after a few days, but occasionally they progressed to very serious infections or hearing loss. Because antibiotics can prevent these complications, office visits and antibiotic prescriptions for ear infections have skyrocketed over the last 40 years. Ear infections are now the most common reason for antibiotic prescription in children. This widespread use of antibiotic drugs for what is usually a self-limiting illness has had the unfortunate result of making the bacteria responsible for ear infections largely resistant to antibiotics, limiting their usefulness.

The issue of antibiotic resistance has caused the medical profession to look much more closely at the way we've been treating ear infections and to make some important changes. We have been ahead of the curve on this one, but since 2004 the treatment guidelines of the AAP echo our antibiotic practices. Since most doctors are still not meeting these guidelines, we need to explain the thinking behind our integrative approach to the common earache.

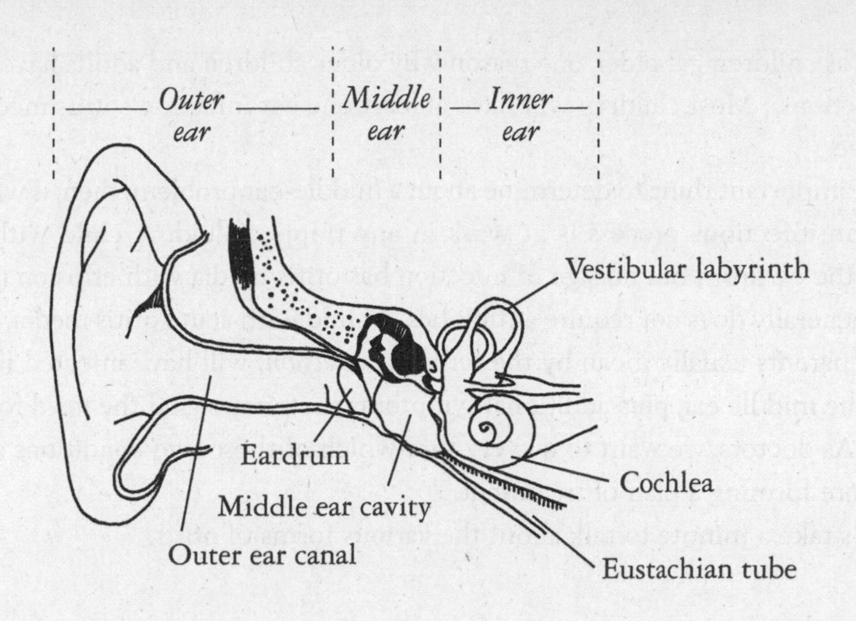

Structures of the Ear

Let's start with a little basic ear anatomy. You are probably already familiar with what is called the outer ear, the shaped cartilage on the side of the head and the ear canal that leads to the eardrum, a tight membrane that transmits sound. The inner ear, which is important to balance, is the portion of the ear located most deeply inside the head, closest to the brain. Between the eardrum and inner ear lies the middle ear, an air-filled cavity that contains three tiny bones essential to hearing. The middle ear is connected to the back of the nasal cavity by the eustachian tube, which provides the air to equalize pressure on both sides of the eardrum. The eustachian tube also allows any fluid produced in the middle ear to drain freely.

You may have already spotted the weak point in this system. Obviously a tube that leads from the back of the nose to the inner ear goes both ways. Not only can fluid drain out of it, but bacteria from the nose or throat can also travel up it. Any obstruction in the tube—a plug of dried mucus, for example—can trap fluid in the middle ear, providing an excellent incubator for stray bacteria. In addition, the eustachian tubes of children under two are more nearly horizontal and more collapsible, so fluid that gets into them cannot easily drain out. (These tubes become more vertical as children get older, one reason why older children and adults have fewer ear infections.) Most children will have at least one ear infection (otitis media) by age three.

The important thing to determine about a middle-ear problem, then, is whether or not an infectious process is at work in any trapped fluid. A child with fluid behind the eardrum but no sign of infection has otitis media with effusion (fluid), which generally does not require antibiotics. A child with acute otitis media, which is what parents usually mean by the term *ear infection*, will have infected fluid or pus in the middle ear, plus additional symptoms that may signal the need for antibiotics. As doctors, we want to be very sure which of these two conditions a child has before forming a plan of treatment.

Let's take a minute to talk about the various forms of otitis.

Problems of the Middle Ear

Otitis Media with Effusion

"Otitis media with effusion" (OME, also called serous OM) is the term we use for times when fluid is present in the middle ear but there is no infection. Symptoms might be a temporary reduction in hearing, a "popping" of the ears, or a feeling of fullness in the ears. Many people—even doctors—confuse fluid in the ear with an ear infection, which is unfortunate, because it leads to about 8 million unnecessary courses of antibiotics a year. The middle ear, like the nose and the sinuses, can collect fluid when a child has a cold or an allergy. Fluid can also be present in the middle ear because of blockage of the eustachian tubes by mucus or enlarged adenoids. In infants, small children, and people with eustachian tube abnormalities, fluid may also be present for weeks or even months after a previous ear infection because of inefficient drainage.

Antibiotics are not prescribed for OME. We monitor kids with OME intermittently and assess the mobility of the eardrum using an instrument called a tympanometer or an air-filled bulb. We want to know whether fluid is starting to drain or getting thicker, and whether hearing is improving or getting worse. If OME persists for more than three months, we refer the child to a pediatric ear, nose, and throat doctor to determine the cause of the fluid. If effusion is especially thick and persistent ("glue ear"), the specialist may recommend the surgical insertion of tiny tubes (discussed in more detail below) to drain the ear.

Acute Otitis Media

"Acute otitis media" (AOM) is what parents typically mean when they talk about an ear infection. It is often distinguished from OME by signs of infection such as fever and reddened eardrums. Older kids may complain of pain or a sensation of fullness in an ear, typically after a cold. Infants who cannot verbalize their pain will be fussy and lack appetite, and may pull or tug at an ear. However, some children with AOM have no fever or pain, and there are many reasons (crying and fever among them) why eardrums might be red when examined by the doctor. To nail down the diagnosis of AOM, your child's doctor needs to use an instrument called an otoscope to examine your child's eardrum. If a child has AOM, her eardrum will bulge outward instead of being in its normal neutral or slightly inward position. It will be opaque (red or yellow), and immobile when air is puffed into the ear canal through a rubber bulb attached to the otoscope.

A bulge in the eardrum is a sign that something nasty is growing in your child's inner ear. Most likely that something is a bacterium (usually *Streptococcus pneumoniae*, *Haemophilus influenzae*, or *Moraxella catarrhalis*). That doesn't necessarily mean that antibiotics are required, a lesson the medical establishment has been slow in learning in this country. One quarter of ear infections are caused by viruses—which we know do not respond to antibiotics—and many of the bacterial cases will get better without any antibiotic drugs. Recent studies have found that 80 percent of cases of AOM caused by *M. catarrhalis* and 50 percent of those caused by *H. influenzae* resolve by themselves within one to seven days. Only 15 to 20 percent of cases caused by *S. pneumoniae* resolve spontaneously, but the pneumonia vaccine can now prevent the majority of those ear infections.

So how do we know when to treat? We prescribe antibiotics from the get-go for a child with an ear infection on both sides, a child with a cleft palate, or a child who is in severe pain, feverish, or fussy, for whom more serious diseases have been ruled out. In most cases of simple AOM where the child is active and alert, however, we prefer a policy of "watchful waiting." That is, we treat the child's ear pain with children's acetaminophen and/or eardrops containing benzocaine (if there is no eardrum rupture). We may also suggest a combination remedy containing extracts of garlic and mullein, which we have found useful. We ask the parents of children under eighteen months to give us a phone report in 24 hours; parents of older children check back with us if the child's fever or pain persists for more than three days. Key to successful watchful waiting are the doctor's correct assessment of the situation, the child's age (older is easier), and the parents' level of reliability.

If there is no sign of improvement, or symptoms worsen, we then prescribe a narrow-spectrum, inexpensive oral antibiotic drug, such as amoxicillin. Often we give a parent a prescription for their child at the first visit and ask them to fill it only if it is still needed after several days. We don't prescribe the newer broad-spectrum antibiotics as a first line of defense but save them for use later if amoxicillin doesn't do the job. These new antibiotics are frequently used unnecessarily, are more expensive, have more side effects, and lead to greater bacterial resistance. When we do prescribe antibiotics, we make sure parents understand that it is important for their child to take these drugs as often and for as long as prescribed. To reduce the risk of diarrhea and other antibiotic side effects, we also strongly suggest that a child eat live-culture yogurt or take probiotic supplements during the course of treatment and for several weeks thereafter.

While it is now supposed to be the standard of practice, this policy of watchful waiting is only gradually gaining support with conventional practitioners as a strategy to slow the rise of resistant bacteria. The bacteria most often responsible for ear infections are increasingly resistant to first-line drug treatment. If doctors focus on saving antibiotics for use only when they are truly clinically appropriate, drug-susceptible strains of these bacteria may be restored. Dr. D has reduced the use of antibiotics in his practice by 60 to 70 percent and is now seeing far fewer cases of recurrent AOM, which can be hard to cure. Dr. Russ's patients in the ED (where follow-up is more difficult) leave knowing that their ear infection will likely go away on its own, but if it doesn't, they have a prescription in hand.

There were once concerns that delaying use of antibiotics for ear infections would lead to serious complications such as the spread of infection to the mastoid area (an air-filled bone directly behind the external ear), brain, or blood. However, studies in the Netherlands, one of the few developed countries where antibiotics are not routinely used for ear infections, found this not to be true. The Dutch practice of watchful waiting has led to a large decline in resistant bacteria in that country.

Sometimes the eardrum bursts spontaneously with sudden pain and discharge of yellowish fluid that may be streaked with red. This relieves pressure (and pain), drains fluid, and allows healing to begin. The eardrum will repair itself naturally. We prescribe oral antibiotics to clear up the infection.

Recurrent AOM

About a quarter of visits to the doctor for ear infection are for acute ear infections that occur three separate times in six months or four or more separate times in a year. Risk factors for recurrent AOM include recent antibiotic use (especially if it was an incomplete course of therapy), age under two years, attendance at a day care center, exposure to tobacco smoke, use of a pacifier, and formula feeding. Underlying conditions such as gastroesophageal reflux, food sensitivities, and enlarged adenoids that serve as a reservoir for bacteria may also play a role and must be treated.

Recurrent cases of AOM are often caused by antibiotic-resistant *S. pneumoniae*, so getting the pneumonia vaccine is an excellent preventive strategy. While the vaccine doesn't yet protect against all strains of pneumonia, it does control the most troublesome ones. Flu vaccines also reduce the number of ear infections experienced. (See chapter 3.)

We treat recurrent AOM with higher doses of amoxicillin or wider-spectrum antibiotics, but we couple that antibiotic approach with an effort to determine and address the underlying problem by recommending the following:

- Try a short trial of a dairy-free diet or other strategies against allergy.
- Support the immune system with rest, nutrition, and fluids.
- Try a daily tonic of the Chinese herb astragalus. Dr. D sometimes advises taking an immune-supportive herbal remedy with echinacea, elderberry, and propolis for up to two weeks.

- See an osteopath or other skilled practitioner for cranial osteopathy or craniosacral manipulation.
- Take a probiotic formula for at least two months following antibiotic therapy.
- Try an anti-reflux medication or send the child to a pediatric ear, nose, and throat specialist for an evaluation for gastroesophageal reflux.

We do not recommend putting children with recurrent AOM on long-term low-dose antibiotics as a preventive measure as this use strongly supports the development of resistant bacteria. We don't jump into it, but if other measures have not been effective and ear infections keep recurring frequently, we consider surgical insertion of pediatric ventilation ear tubes in the eardrums. Although the invasive procedure requires general anesthesia, it is usually quite safe, even for infants. A child with tubes will have to wear earplugs for swimming afterward, but the middle ear will be able to drain more freely, and there will be less scarring than from repeated rupture. Eventually your child will outgrow the need for tubes, which usually fall out naturally on their own within a year or two, allowing the eardrum to heal over.

Problems of the Outer Ear

Otitis Externa ("Swimmer's Ear")

As opposed to otitis media, otitis externa is an inflammation of the outer ear canal, usually seen in the summer months. It's not caused by the same bacteria as acute otitis media, but rather by inflammatory conditions of the skin, by trauma, or by organisms such as *Pseudomonas, Staphylococcus aureus*, and various fungi that get too comfy in the moist environment of the ear canal. In children, otitis externa can cause itching, discharge, and pain but has no serious complications. (As the same symptoms present when your child has put a bean in his ear, check for foreign objects first.)

We take a two-pronged approach to otitis externa:

- Preventive eardrops of equal parts alcohol and white vinegar to restore the acid pH of the ear canal and prevent their return. Just put a few drops of this solution into each ear, especially after swimming. Earplugs can be helpful while swimming too.
- Prescription antibiotic eardrops to kill off infecting organisms.

Preventing Ear Infections

- Avoid exposing your child to tobacco smoke. Children of smokers have more ear infections.
- Breast-feed your child, if possible. Infants who have been breast-fed at least three or four months have fewer ear infections.
- Don't feed infants in a flat position or give a baby a bottle to take into the crib. (Remember our description of the anatomy of the ear?)
- Limit the use of a pacifier to just a few minutes at bedtime. Better yet, don't use one at all.
- Encourage frequent hand washing, especially before snacks or meals.
- Teach your child to blow her nose gently and without pinching her nostrils together to avoid shooting that gunk up into her middle ear.
- Consider a smaller day care situation if your child has recurrent ear infections.
- Children who are sensitive to milk proteins can develop increased irritation and inflammation in the upper airway. Try eliminating dairy products from your child's diet for a month or two if he has recurrent ear infections. (Be sure to provide adequate calcium from other foods or supplements.)
- Consider dietary supplements that might help prevent recurrent infections. Dr. D has seen good results from essential fatty acids and from both garlic and elderberry extracts.
- Vaccinate with Prevnar against *Streptococcus pneumoniae*, which causes

20 percent of ear infections and accounts for many cases of recurrent AOM.

▶ Consider cranial osteopathy. Birth trauma and minor childhood accidents may increase susceptibility to ear infections by restricting the free flow of fluids in the head. Dr. Russ has heard reports of recurrent ear infections resolving from this treatment.

Treating Ear Infections

▶ Use children's acetaminophen and anesthetic eardrops for pain relief. Never use pain-relieving or herbal eardrops when there is discharge of blood or pus from the ear.

▶ Use antibiotics properly. Don't pressure the physician for the drugs, but if they are prescribed, make sure your child takes all the pills or liquid as ordered and takes a probiotic supplement during and for two weeks after treatment.

▶ Apply gentle heat to the ear with a warm compress.

▶ Put 2 or 3 drops of garlic oil or garlic-mullein oil in the ear several times a day and plug loosely with a little cotton. Don't put drops in any ear with suspected rupture of the eardrum. This is Dr. D's approach, and he sometimes supplements this topical treatment with garlic taken orally as food or supplement.

▶ Echinacea can sometimes be helpful at the start of an ear infection

▶ Try a homeopathic remedy that suits your child's symptoms, preferences, and temperament. Possibilities include *Aconite, Apis, Belladonna, Capsicum, Chamomilla, Kali bichromate, Mercurius, Silica*, and *Pulsatilla*.

As a final note on earaches, keep in mind that not all earaches are actually caused by ear infections. Other causes of ear pain include an abscessed tooth, a sinus infection, a sore throat (pharyngitis), and temperomandibular joint syndrome (TMJ), and these conditions will need to be ruled out.

CHAPTER 17

Colic and Reflux

It's the middle of the night, and six-week-old Max has been screaming at the top of his lungs for hours. His exhausted parents are nearly in tears themselves from their inability to comfort their tightly wound child. Finally his dad throws a coat over his pajamas, wraps up the red-faced Max, and heads for the car. He'll drive his little boy around for a few hours, the only thing that ever seems to soothe him.

Dramas like this are played out in households around the country, though the makeshift solutions to a colicky child vary. We've heard of kids soothed by driving, by the sound of a washer/dryer, and by the touch of massage. We know how exhausting and stressful colic can be for both parents and child. And we know how difficult it can be to build that essential parent-child bond when parents feel helpless and frustrated by their inability to provide comfort.

When dealing with an irritable baby, colic is the diagnosis we make when more serious problems have been ruled out. Colic is not a specific disease with a set cause but rather a group of behaviors that occur in about 20 percent of infants in their first few months of life. Babies are considered to have colic if they:

- Cry intensely for three or more hours a day at least three days a week and do not have any obvious physical reason for the crying

- Scream for longer periods of time than average children and are more difficult to console
- Are irritable and frequently have difficulty relaxing
- Feed well despite these symptoms

Infantile colic occurs at about the same time of day or night, most often night. It usually appears at about two weeks of age, peaks at six weeks, and disappears when the child is three to four months old. If "colic" continues for longer or involves poor feeding and crying during or after feedings, it is probably actually reflux, which we'll discuss below. Colic has no adverse long-term effects.

Despite any number of theories, no single cause of colic has been identified. Factors such as food allergies or intolerances, abdominal pain, intestinal gas, and difficult parent-child relationships have all been studied and dismissed as overall causes, although each can contribute to the symptoms of colic. Current research leans toward colic being either a neurodevelopmental stage in certain children who are extremely sensitive to their environments or an immaturity of the gastrointestinal tract that only time can cure.

While we don't know much about the cause of colic, we do know that infantile colic will go away with time. In the meanwhile, parents need to experiment until they find a few comfortable positions or soothing behaviors that calm their child. Once you have a few trusty tools, plan to use them as soon as possible after crying starts, as it is easier to relax a child who is not yet totally wound up.

Take care of yourselves too, as colic can give parents an extremely stressful few months. Make sure you have some release valve, a good friend or an emergency child-care site, to which you can turn if sleep deprivation and frustration lead you to think about shaking or hurting your child. There's no shame in asking for help when you and your child need it. Colicky babies can wear out even the most durable parents over time, if parents do not take the time-outs they need to regroup.

How to Deal with Colic

There is no disease process to arrest with colic, so we target our treatment to the symptoms. In our experience, over-the-counter colic remedies containing simethicone aren't effective, but the nine strategies below have been helpful to our patients and our own kids. Because every child is unique, we cannot predict what strategies will work for your child. Some babies need the stimulation of sound, motion, or touch. Others are soothed by calm, quiet surroundings. Every baby has an "off" switch; you'll have to experiment to find what triggers your child's.

1. *Try a gentle massage for up to fifteen minutes once or twice a day*. This is a simple and effective way to reduce the pain and tension of both colicky baby and parents. Use a palmful of moisturizing baby cream or lotion.

2. *Give a bottle of up to four ounces a day of warm (not hot) herbal chamomile or fennel tea*. This can soothe an irritable baby for several hours.

3. *Lower your anxiety level*. Nervous or agitated parents aggravate regurgitation in babies. Choose and practice whatever form of stress reduction works best for you in order to prevent a vicious cycle of irritation between parent and baby.

4. *Try some lavender aromatherapy*. Use a little sedative lavender oil in a diffuser in baby's room. We don't recommend regular massage with lavender oil, as the herb appears to have estrogenic effects when used on infant skin.

5. *Keep that baby moving*. Rock or roll your baby in a rhythmic and relaxed manner. Put him in a sling or a front- or backpack and go for a walk. Drive aimlessly around in the car trying not to feel guilty about the fossil fuels you're burning.

6. *Try white noise*. Turn on the washer/dryer or the vacuum cleaner in the next room. Put on a tape of a mother's heartbeat, ocean waves, or lullabies.

7. *Assume the position*. Some positions are better than others at soothing

a colicky child. One of the classics is the "flying baby" or "sack of potatoes" pose, with infant draped, stomach down, along a parent's forearm.

8. *Swaddle the baby*. Some babies like to have their bodies wrapped snugly (face free) in a sheet or blanket.

9. *Experiment with alternative medicine*. Some parents swear by cranial osteopathy for colic. Others say homeopathic remedies have done the trick.

Call your child's physician immediately if your child has persistent or rapid-fire vomiting, fever, lethargy, refusal to feed, or is inconsolable.

But what if it's not just colic? There is another condition that is often confused with colic in young children: *gastroesophageal reflux*, or *reflux*. Reflux is most familiar to adults as the "heartburn" caused by acidic stomach contents backing up into the esophagus. Infants may experience heartburn and abdominal pain with reflux as well, but their primary symptom is often frequent or recurrent spitting up. In some cases the stomach secretions rise high enough to irritate and inflame the upper and lower airways (nose, throat, and bronchial tubes) and may even lead to chronic respiratory infections, cough, sinusitis, ear infections, congestion, or the wheezing of reactive airways.

How can you tell colic from reflux? A baby more likely has reflux if she spits up frequently or if her symptoms last longer than three months. Some infants with reflux (known as "happy spitters") eat well and spit up without pain. Others have pain associated with their vomiting. Some of the sickest and most uncomfortable babies with reflux, however, never spit up at all.

That's why doctors and parents should pay attention to feeding patterns. Usually, healthy babies look forward to and enjoy feeding times. Babies with colic may initially resist feeding but eventually will relax and feed. Most babies with reflux, however, find it difficult to relax with feeding and often refuse to feed because doing so aggravates the burning sensation ("heartburn") in the esophagus. They arch their backs in a certain way and appear uncomfortable in their own skin. Babies with reflux may exhibit pain for one or two hours after feeding, and some may develop anticipatory pain before feeding or just from smelling milk.

more on . . .

HAPPY SPITTERS AND PAINFUL SPITTERS

In happy spitters, immaturity of the muscle that closes the lower esophagus during digestion causes partially digested food or milk to escape the stomach and move painlessly toward the outside world. Put them on their backs at a 45-degree angle after feedings, and they'll be fine. Painful spitters, on the other hand, have a problem with an overly acid stomach that makes feeding painful. Treatment for painful spitters may be a change in mom's diet, a change in formula, or a prescription antacid.

Although older children with reflux may also have heartburn or stomachache, reflux is more likely to appear in kids over three as frequent upper respiratory infections, reactive airway disease, hoarseness, or ear infections. In our experience, treating the underlying problem of reflux can eradicate these persistent conditions. Successful treatment of reflux may also eliminate the need for long-term antibiotics to treat recurrent ear and sinus infections.

Simple reflux tends to clear up on its own by the time a child is walking (twelve to fifteen months). But untreated chronic reflux (gastroesophageal reflux disease, or GERD) can cause serious discomfort, so we try to diagnose and treat it in a timely manner.

Take your child to the emergency department immediately if reflux is accompanied by breathing difficulties, wheezing, frequent coughing, turning blue, or brief periods of not breathing (apnea).

How to Deal with Reflux

Once your child's doctor has diagnosed reflux, there are remedies that can be employed by both parent and physician. Among them:

- *Change the child's diet.* Food sensitivities can play a role in reflux. Sensitivity to breast milk is extremely rare, so we strongly recommend breastfeeding for babies with reflux. If reflux continues, mother may need to eliminate cow's milk from her own diet. If that doesn't do the trick, then she should try an elimination diet (see chapter 20) to identify possible dietary allergens. Babies being fed formula based on cow's milk should be switched to a hydrolyzed casein- or soy-based formula. If these are ineffective, try a hypoallergenic predigested protein hydrolysate formula such as Nutramigen, Alimentum, or Good Start.

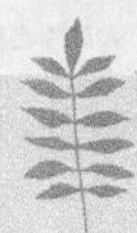

TIP: Older children with reflux should avoid chocolate, caffeine, peppermint, and carbonated beverages, any of which can trigger esophageal reflux because they relax the muscle that seals the stomach off from the esophagus.

▶ *Consider the child's position.* Babies with reflux may feel better if they're placed in an infant seat at a 45-degree angle for a short time after feeding.

▶ *Thicken feedings.* Add a tablespoon of rice cereal to each ounce of formula to reduce regurgitation in bottle-fed babies. This increases calories per ounce from 20 to 30, so families where weight gain is an issue should look for special prethickened formulas that deliver just the desired 20 calories per ounce.

▶ *Try a prescription medication.* When a child is in significant pain—especially while feeding—and not eating an adequate number of calories, we often prescribe a drug such as ranitidine (Zantac) or lansoprazole (Prevacid) to reduce or neutralize stomach acid, ease burning, and allow the esophagus to heal.

▶ *Avoid tobacco.* Exposure to tobacco smoke worsens reflux in babies.

▶ *Try probiotics for at least two months.* Either add to formula or "paint" a slurry of probiotic powder and water onto mother's nipple before breastfeeding.

▶ *Focus on relaxing yourself.* Like colic, reflux is aggravated by parental anxiety. Take time-outs when you need them, and practice deep breathing or some other stress-busting technique.

CHAPTER 18

Tummy Troubles

The belly seems to be the focus of many pediatric complaints. We see lots of kids with "school-day tummy pain," constipation, and diarrhea, as well as kids with more serious gastrointestinal disorders. One reason why the abdomen is the site of so much trouble is that the belly is where children tend to carry stress from worrying or unresolved conflicts. Even so, parents should not jump to the conclusion that tummy trouble is always stress related. There are about a hundred possible causes of abdominal pain, from self-limiting illnesses to problems requiring surgery, so it's essential to come up with the right diagnosis. In the following pages, we'll discuss some of the most common causes of tummy troubles we see in children and our recommendations for treatment.

Constipation

A child is considered constipated if she is moving her bowels fewer than three times a week, is straining or having painful voiding, or is passing hard, dry stools. Many children have problems with constipation at some time in their young lives, most often from lack of fluids, poor diet, or withholding of stool either for psychological reasons or due to pain while defecating. Kids may hold stool when they are being toilet trained or if they are uncomfortable using a bathroom not their own.

In our experience, parents have a tendency to get worked up about a possibly constipated child, so we counsel you to try to project a more relaxed attitude. You don't want this to become a battle of wills. Among the suggestions below, you will find a number of strategies for relieving constipation that can be instituted without a child's really being conscious of them. We do not generally use artificial laxatives for children with constipation, preferring gentler, more natural methods. In cases of long-term constipation, however, we may resort to intermittent use of mild laxatives or stool softeners, or a pediatric enema.

Constipation can be a contributing factor in recurrent urinary infections, especially in girls, as the free flow of urine is blocked by impacted stool. *Call your child's doctor* for any constipation that does not resolve with time, as it can be the sign of a more serious problem.

Dealing with Constipation

- *Assess your child's milk consumption.* We often see constipation in toddlers who drink more than two cups of cow's milk a day. If cow's milk is identified as a problem after elimination from the diet for a trial period, switch to calcium-fortified soy milk.

- *Make sure your child is drinking enough fluids.* Children should drink a cup of water a day for every ten pounds of weight (up to eighty pounds).

- *Increase physical activity.* Regular exercise helps keep things moving along, intestinally speaking.

- *Increase fiber consumption.* Make sure your child eats plenty of high-fiber foods such as fruits, vegetables, whole-grain bread, bran flakes, beans, and brown rice.

- *Try some prunes.* Grandma was right! A few tablespoons a day of stewed prunes for babies, or three to four stewed or dried prunes a day for toddlers can help keep them regular.

- *Add probiotics*. Beneficial bacteria, such as lactobacilli or bifidobacteria, may help, either in the form of yogurt with live cultures, kefir, or supplements. These "good bugs" certainly help with digestion, and some studies have found benefit for constipation as well.

- *Bulk up*. We recommend two high-fiber natural laxatives, flax and psyllium. Dr. D prefers ground flaxseed meal, which has a mild and nutty flavor and the added benefit of omega-3 fatty acids. (Whole, unground flaxseeds can actually worsen constipation.) Give a child over age two a teaspoon a day of flaxseed meal sprinkled over his food; adjust the dose up or down as needed. Keep flaxseeds or meal frozen or refrigerated, as flax products turn rancid quickly when exposed to air and light. (Discard any flax product that smells like paint, a sure sign of rancidity.)

  Dr. Russ usually suggests either a teaspoon of powdered psyllium seed husks (*Plantago psyllium*) a day or a mix of the powdered husks and flax meal. The psyllium should be stirred into a large glass of juice or water and drunk. A child taking either of these natural laxatives should be sure to drink plenty of water and other fluids throughout the day, otherwise these "bulking agents" will just plug things up worse.

- *Check out emotional issues*. Withholding stool can be a form of control, or a sign of stress. Be sure not to be punitive during toilet training or to reprimand a child for bowel accidents or constipation; you'll only worsen the situation. Allow for a relaxed regular "sit-down" period for your child. Self-hypnosis, meditation, biofeedback, or breathing exercises may be helpful for general stress reduction.

Diarrhea

Diarrhea is a condition of loose, frequent stools, often accompanied by a feeling of "gotta go." While diarrheal illness is one of the leading causes of infant death in developing countries, here in the United States, diarrhea is usually due to a mild, self-limiting infection.

Diarrhea is most commonly due to viruses, bacteria, or parasites picked up from other kids, contaminated water, or improperly prepared foods. One simple preventive strategy to reduce exposure to these infectious agents is teaching your children to wash their hands carefully after going the bathroom and before preparing or eating food. When traveling in developing countries, don't let them drink or brush their teeth with any water that is not purified, or eat food from street vendors. Failure to follow these simple rules can lead to a vacation-spoiling case of "travelers' diarrhea." At home, "food poisoning" caused by such microbes as *Salmonella* and *E. coli* can often be quite severe, so be sure to handle, prepare, and store food safely. Don't let your child eat raw cookie dough or other foods containing undercooked meat or eggs.

So-called "antibiotic-associated diarrhea" is the frequent result of treatment with antibiotics that wipe out beneficial bowel bacteria as a side effect. Use of probiotics should prevent this.

Call your child's physician if diarrhea is accompanied by cramping pain, fever, or bloody stools; if a nonpainful case of diarrhea continues for more than five days; or if persistent diarrhea follows a camping trip or travel in a developing country.

Take your child to the doctor or emergency department immediately if he exhibits signs of dehydration such as sunken eyes or "doughy" skin, or refuses to take in fluids.

Dealing with Diarrhea

▶ *Give your child plenty of liquids.* Best here is an electrolyte-balanced drink or popsicle. Plain water can actually dilute salt and contribute to electrolyte imbalance in a very young child. Avoid high-sugar fruit juices or sodas.

▶ *Give a probiotic supplement.* We recommend that any child who has had diarrhea for more than two or three days be given supplemental probiotics for seven to ten days. If a child is too young to swallow an enteric-coated probiotic capsule, sprinkle probiotic powder or the contents of a probiotic capsule on food or put it in formula.

▶ *If diarrhea persists, consider reducing or eliminating milk products from your child's diet.* Many children have an allergy or sensitivity to a milk protein called casein. Others—especially those of African American, Asian, or Mediterranean heritage—lack the enzyme lactase, which is necessary to digest a milk sugar called lactose. Even children who normally can digest milk well may experience a temporary lactase deficiency while ill, resulting in diarrhea.

- *A bland diet gives the intestines time to regroup*. Aptly called BRAT, the conventional diet includes bananas, rice, applesauce, and dry toast. We add yogurt as well after the first day of a diarrheal illness.

We discourage the use of over-the-counter diarrhea remedies as they slow down the peristaltic activity of the gut so that it takes longer for a child's body to get rid of any pathogens. This is especially important with bacterial causes of diarrhea.

Inflammatory Bowel Disease

Whenever a child has persistent abdominal pain, unexplained recurrent fever, and bloody diarrhea, we need to consider *inflammatory bowel disease*, or IBD. This term encompasses both Crohn's disease and ulcerative colitis, conditions that are sometimes difficult to distinguish from one another. A diagnosis of IBD is made after an extensive history and physical exam, tests for inflammation or infection (such as blood test of sedimentation rate and the presence of specific IBD antibodies), and perhaps a barium X-ray or direct visual evaluation of the bowel through endoscopy.

IBD is usually treated with strong anti-inflammatory drugs that can have significant side effects. We have had great success with drug-free strategies, which, although they do require a great commitment from child and parents, can stop diarrhea, pain, and bleeding and help a child regain lost weight.

The foundation of Dr. D's IBD treatment is a dietary program designed by nutritionist Elaine Gottschall (see Resources), which, after a period of close monitoring, has allowed many of his patients to avoid immunosuppressive therapy. Although her IBD diet is quite restrictive—eliminating all cereal grains and (liquid) milk—highly motivated children and families have found it well worth the inconvenience to be free of their disabling symptoms. Dr. D allows some modifications to the Gottschall program, but, in his experience, it works best when followed strictly.

Dr. Russ takes a more individualized tack with his patients, using food-elimination trials to help pinpoint their unique IBD triggers. He has found that this approach provides symptomatic relief while minimizing dietary restrictions.

The cause of IBD is not really known, though we do know that stress is an important factor. Therefore, both of us rely heavily on mind/body therapies as well, including relaxation techniques, biofeedback, and imagery.

Dealing with IBD

- *Try an elimination diet*. This will help pinpoint foods that worsen your child's symptoms, and should be avoided.

- *Help your child learn and practice a suitable stress-reduction technique*.

- *Boost your child's intake of anti-inflammatory omega-3 fatty acids*. Try either food (cold-water fish) or fish oil supplements at a dose of 1 to 2 g a day for children under twelve.

- *Try acupuncture*. A number of Dr. Russ's patients have experienced good results from this complementary approach.

- *Cut out caffeinated soft drinks*.

- *Consider enteric-coated peppermint oil capsules for children old enough to swallow*. Do not substitute any other form of peppermint oil, which in its raw form can cause young children to choke. Don't use peppermint in children with gastroesophageal reflux.

- *Consider probiotics*. We've seen promising research data and anecdotal evidence of its benefit in IBD.

Celiac Disease

Celiac disease (celiac sprue) is an autoimmune disorder caused by an inherited inability to digest gluten, a protein found in many common grains. The undigested gluten causes inflammation in the small intestine that can lead to permanent damage. Symptoms include diarrhea, abdominal pain, bloating, rumbling of the gut, and weight loss. Consider celiac disease in a preteen who is growing poorly or a teen slow to develop secondary sexual characteristics.

Celiac disease can usually be diagnosed by a simple blood test. People with celiac disease must avoid or limit foods containing wheat, barley, rye, spelt, kamut, and possibly oats, and many processed foods containing products made from these grains. Fortunately most supermarkets now carry gluten-free products.

Functional Abdominal Pain

Functional abdominal pain is how doctors describe pain around the belly button with no known organic cause. The fact that there is no physical reason for the pain does not mean that the pain is not real, and even debilitating. As we all know, stress can play a lot of nasty tricks on us. But once all the serious diseases have been ruled out, it's almost a relief to know that your child's pain can be controlled or eliminated without drugs or surgery.

Most parents are familiar with the kind of belly pain we're talking about. This is the before-school or bedtime pain, the pain that appears at school or in the doctor's office, or wherever a stressful situation can be found. It's the pain of fear and anxiety and conflicted feelings. It's a pain that goes away when a child is having a good time or feeling relaxed and comforted. And don't underestimate the power of parental comfort and reassurance. In our experience, kids with functional abdominal pain will not be themselves relieved until their parents are reassured that this is a correct diagnosis.

In order to provide this reassurance, we do a complete workup to rule out serious disorders, which are more likely if fever, nausea, vomiting, painful urination, weight loss, or bloody stools are involved. We put the emphasis on talking to the child and to his parents about his social circumstances—his relationships with school, friends, and family—looking for sources of stress. Sometimes an apprehensive child simply needs to know that all tests are normal for the pain to disappear. Other times we will need to have an open discussion with child and parents about the connection between their stress and their pain and work together to create a program to manage and eliminate the source of stress. We may refer a family to a therapist to work on those deeper issues.

A more chronic form of functional abdominal pain is *irritable bowel syndrome* (IBS), whose symptoms also include bloating, cramping, and either diarrhea or constipation, or a mix of both. The cause of IBS has been hard to pin down, because testing only reveals a normal bowel. We do know that in most cases stress worsens the symptoms of IBS considerably, perhaps because so much of the body's supply of serotonin is found in the bowel. We generally turn to dietary manipulation and mind/body therapies such as stress management and self-hypnosis to deal with the underlying causes. A series of food eliminations may uncover any allergies or intolerances, and both probiotics and traditional Chinese medicine may help soothe an irritated bowel.

Helicobacter pylori Infection

A majority of children carry the bacterium *Helicobacter pylori* in their stomachs, apparently without problem. However, lifestyle factors such as stress, poor diet, or weakened immunity may render a child more vulnerable to the bacterium's effects. The end result may be an infection of the upper gastrointestinal tract that causes pain in the upper belly and sometimes nausea, burping, and vomiting. The infection usually resolves on its own, but when symptoms are severe or resistant to the integrative treatments below, we prescribe a regimen of two antibiotics and an acid reducer, with a side dose of probiotics.

Dealing with *H. pylori*

- *Have your child practice a mind/body therapy for stress reduction.* Studies have tied an inability to cope with stress to an increase in stomach acid secretions and a worsening of ulcer symptoms.
- *Try an herbal extract called deglycyrrhizinated licorice (DGL).* This soothes the stomach and duodenum and supports natural defenses. It's available in

tablets that can be chewed and swallowed whenever the child feels discomfort. The only catch is that he has to like the taste of licorice. (Most candies don't contain real licorice and will not do the trick. In any case, you do not want to give a child extracts or other forms of licorice containing glycyrrhizin, as the compound raises blood pressure.)

▶ *Avoid soft drinks, especially caffeinated ones*. Try warm or iced chamomile or peppermint tea instead. (Kids with GERD should avoid peppermint.)

▶ *Reduce inflammation naturally*. Dr. D, as you may have noticed, is a big fan of ginger, so he suggests experimenting to see if taking (or eating) ginger eases symptoms. Ginger also contains some compounds specifically effective against ulcer.

Appendicitis

Whenever a child has persistent abdominal pain it is important to rule out *appendicitis*. Acute inflammation of this little dead-end tube off the large intestine can become a life-threatening condition. If an untreated "hot" appendix is not surgically removed in time, it can burst, spreading infection throughout the abdominal cavity.

Whenever we see a child with progressive abdominal pain we do a thorough physical exam, some basic lab tests if they are clinically indicated, and possibly a follow-up imaging study (sonogram or CT scan), because we want to be very careful not to miss a case of appendicitis. Most children with appendicitis will have vomiting and loss of appetite in addition to the abdominal pain. They may not eat for two or three days. Very young children cannot describe their pain verbally, but in older children, pain is generalized or starts around the belly button, and gradually localizes in the lower right part of the abdomen over the ensuing hours. The cure for appendicitis is strictly surgical—remove the inflamed appendix—and recovery is generally uneventful. (Be sure that strep throat has been ruled out before an appendectomy, as strep throat can, oddly, also cause abdominal pain that can be mistaken for appendicitis.)

CHAPTER 19

Headache

A pounding head might seem to be an adult problem, but kids get headaches too. In fact, 40 percent of children suffer at least one headache before the age of seven. A child's headaches can stem from a wide array of causes: dehydration, noise, glaring light, a skipped meal, exposure to chemicals, vision problems, stress, head injuries, and such medical conditions as fever, strep throat, sinus infection, meningitis, misalignment of the jaw, and yes, brain tumor. In order to treat a headache, and prevent future headaches, you and your child's physician need to figure out what factor or combination of factors is behind your child's headaches. In this chapter, we talk about the two most common forms of headache in children, tension and migraine, and briefly touch on temporomandibular joint syndrome (TMJ), which can also cause head pain.

See your child's physician or *take your child to the emergency department* if a headache was caused by a fall or head injury, if it involves seizure, lethargy, vomiting, clumsiness, or personality changes, or if it worsens over a period of days. Parents often think that a child who has sustained a fall should not be allowed to go to sleep for fear they'll lapse into a coma. In fact, a little nap can help ease the trauma; just wake the child up in an hour.

TIP: Carbon monoxide poisoning is a serious and common cause of headache and flu-like symptoms, especially in the winter months when gas furnaces, space heaters, and generators are in greater use. Make sure heaters are in good working order and used in well-ventilated areas. Don't let children be in a closed garage when car, lawn mower, or go-cart engines are running.

Tension Headaches

The main symptom of tension headache is a dull pain that affects the whole head. It can feel like a tight band around the skull or a generalized achiness. The cause of this common headache is usually physical or mental stress, which tightens up the muscles of the head, neck, and shoulders.

The best approach to stress-related problems is twofold—ease the symptoms (short-term relief) and try to get at the root of the problem (long-term relief). If your child is experiencing recurrent tension-type headaches, a gentle exploratory conversation may be in order. Often children will try to hide concerns or emotions that they—rightly or wrongly—believe will add to their parents' own stress levels. Speaking freely about what's bothering them can go a long way toward easing stress-related headaches. It's important that they learn that a tension headache is a message, a signal from the body that it's time to stop and take care of yourself.

TIP: Pay attention to your own tension headaches, noting when and why they occur, and what therapies or lifestyle changes make them disappear. Then, if you see similar signs of tension headaches in your children, you'll have some useful tips to pass along.

Dealing with a Tension Headache

As we said before, there are many possible causes of headache, so first make sure your child has had enough sleep, enough food, and enough water that day. Ask about any minor accidents that involved the head, and check for the presence of fever or infection. If you've spoken with your doctor and ruled out these causes, consider strategies that address tension.

▶ *Figure out the cause of tension.* Has your child had an argument with her best friend? Is she worried about an upcoming test or performance? Is there tension within the family that needs to be addressed? Talk with your child about what's going on in her life. If the problem is either severe or long-standing, and does not respond to treatment, your child's doctor may suggest a visit to a psychologist or therapist for further help.

▶ *Use a relaxation, self-hypnosis, or visualization exercise to help your child reduce body tension.* See the sample exercise in the box on page 259.

▶ *Try an acupressure self-care technique.* Press gently with the tips of the middle fingers in the two depressions at the base of the skull on either side of the spine for a few minutes. Pressing with one thumb on the highest point of the muscle in the webbing between the other thumb and forefinger may also help with headache pain. If a complete examination by your child's doctor has ruled out other physical causes for persistent headaches, you could also consult a licensed acupuncturist for instruction in specific acupressure point therapy for headaches, or for acupuncture for older children.

▶ *Keep a headache diary.* If headaches become frequent, make note of the activities of the day, foods eaten, worries, etc. See if you can detect a pattern that helps unlock the cause. If the headaches seem to be tied to certain foods or food additives, pinpoint problems using a food-elimination trial as explained in the next chapter.

▶ *Gently massage your child's head, shoulders, and neck.* Give special attention to the areas above and in front of the ears.

▶ *Take your child on a walk or suggest some other exercise to release tension.*

▶ *Encourage your child to do something he loves.* This provides distraction and stress relief.

▶ *Try a homeopathic remedy, such as* Gelsemium *or* Natrum muriaticum.

▶ *Apply heat or cold, depending on personal preference.* Apply ice or a bag of frozen corn wrapped in a light towel, or either warm (test it on your own skin first) or cold compresses to the forehead or back of the neck.

▶ *Give your child an age-appropriate dose of over-the-counter pain reliever, such as acetaminophen or ibuprofen.*

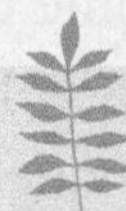

TIP: Dehydration is a common cause of headache in children, especially during school days. Encourage your kids to keep sipping water throughout the day.

Temporomandibular Joint Syndrome

Misalignment of the joint where the jaw meets the skull (the temporomandibular joint) is a common cause for head pain in both children and adults. *Temporomandibular joint syndrome* (TMJ) can have its roots in an accident or sports injury, in misaligned teeth, or in tension or spasm that pulls the muscles and other structures of the mid-lower face out of place. We consider the stress-related form of TMJ as a more severe form of tension headache with slightly different symptoms. A child with TMJ might have pain radiating to one ear, difficulty chewing, loss of appetite, and/or headache. She might grind her teeth at night (bruxism). Mind/body techniques or a nighttime dental appliance can relax the muscles and stabilize the joint. There may be benefit from osteopathic cranial manipulation or acupuncture as well. Any therapies should be coordinated with orthodontic assessment and treatment as needed.

Migraine Headaches

Many parents are surprised to hear that even infants as young as six months of age can get migraines, but these disabling headaches are actually the most common type in children. *Migraines* come in many forms. A migraine can give a child the same throbbing headache, dizziness, and sensitivity to light and noise typical to adult sufferers. In children, oddly, a migraine is even more often associated with gastrointestinal symptoms such as nausea, vomiting, and abdominal pain. Migraines can also present in bizarre ways, such as confusion, temporary memory loss, and stroke-like symptoms. The migraines of children are generally shorter in duration than those of adults, bilateral rather than one-sided, and lasting from ten to fifteen minutes to a few hours rather than lingering for days. They may worsen during puberty as a result of hormonal changes.

There is a very strong genetic component to migraine that gives some people sensitive nervous systems that react more strongly to stimulation. Nearly half of kids with a parent who gets migraines will get them too. The exact sequence of events in migraine is still a mystery, but we do know that this type of headache is often triggered by foods, activities, odors, menstruation, and the environment. Triggers vary from person to person, but common ones include hot dogs and cold cuts, aged cheese, chocolate, bananas, caffeine, foods containing MSG or nitrites, stress, glaring light, hunger, noise, weather changes, and lack of sleep. Some people react to just one trigger; others will need to have several of them occur at once to get a migraine. A kid with a history of migraines who stays up late, sloshes down several cola drinks, and skips breakfast in the morning may be setting herself up for a migraine attack.

Migraine headaches are divided into two categories based on the absence or presence of a warning stage called the *aura*. Most people have what is called a migraine without aura, or *common migraine*, but some experience migraine with aura, or *classical migraine*. Up to two days before a migraine begins, children may show physical or emotional symptoms such as pale skin, fatigue, food cravings, irritability, or hyperactivity (prodrome). If they have classical migraine, there may be a period of up to an hour of visual disturbances like flashing lights or zigzags that fade as the headache kicks in (aura). Once you and your child have talked about these early symptoms and are aware of their meaning, you can use them as cues to start preventive measures to abort or lessen an attack.

There are some migraine drugs for adults that might be of use in children with severe migraines, although most have not been tested in children and can have significant side effects. So rather than prescribe dihydroergotamine, beta blockers, or sumatriptan alone for migraine, we prefer to start with noninvasive approaches, such as elimination of triggers and use of mind/body techniques for symptom control.

A VISUALIZATION EXERCISE FOR HEADACHE PAIN

Sit comfortably and breathe slowly, deeply, and evenly. Imagine that healing energy is pouring over your head like warm sunshine. As it pours down your body, it makes you feel looser–like your arms and legs are made of Jell-O. As you relax, imagine yourself in a fun place or doing something you love. Imagine all the beautiful colors, smells, textures, and sounds as you create this picture or movie in your mind. As you continue to breathe slowly and deeply, enjoy the picture and remember how good you feel when you are in that special place or doing that special activity. Imagine your pain melting away as you enjoy yourself.

Dealing with Migraine Headaches

▶ *Keep a migraine diary*. The best approach for reducing the frequency of migraines is to identify your child's triggers. Keep track of weather, diet, and other possible factors in a migraine diary, analyzing this information yourself or with your child's doctor and avoiding, eliminating, or at least preparing for those factors that seem to be potential triggers. We see the best outcomes when a child takes an active role, so let your child take the lead here.

▶ *Make sure your child is getting enough sleep and not missing a meal*. Missing a meal is a trigger for 25 percent of kids with migraine. Not drinking enough water can also be a trigger, especially in active toddlers.

▶ *Teach your child a mind/body technique for self-regulation*. Therapies such as biofeedback and self-hypnosis are among the most effective interventions for children with headaches. A few sessions with a specialist and some practice will prepare your child ahead of time to deal with the symptoms of migraine. Older kids might benefit from exposure to mindfulness meditation and yoga (no inverted postures), with a special emphasis on breathing exercises.

▶ *Allow the child to rest in a dark, quiet room*. Most children will react to the sudden onset of a migraine by wanting to go to bed. Let them follow their instincts here—rest or sleep can completely relieve a migraine attack.

Talk to your child's teacher about allowing him to put his head down and rest if a migraine starts in school.

▶ *Use heat or cold*. Microwaved hot packs or freezer cold packs may help relieve symptoms. See which one your child prefers. Test hot packs on yourself first, and put a cloth between a cold pack and your child's skin.

▶ *Eliminate artificial ingredients*. Migraine attacks can be triggered by processed foods with such additives as nitrites, MSG, aspartame (Nutrasweet), or caffeine.

▶ *Cut saturated fats and increase anti-inflammatory omega-3 fatty acids in your child's diet*. This can be accomplished through intake of cold-water fish, ground flaxseed, or fish oil supplements.

▶ *Relieve pain with children's acetaminophen or ibuprofen*. Use as directed for up to two days. If symptoms persist longer, consult your child's doctor. Stronger prescription pain relievers are available, but they have not been tested in children and do have side effects.

▶ *Consider a visit to a homeopath for an acute or constitutional remedy to reduce migraines*. Homeopathic (not herbal) *Belladonna*, *Iris*, and *Sanguinaria* are common remedies for migraine, based on specific characteristics.

▶ *Give acupuncture or cranial osteopathy a trial*. Dr. Russ has witnessed excellent results from these two therapies in children who had already been through conventional Western medical evaluation to rule out more serious conditions.

▶ *Try a botanical remedy*. The natural anti-inflammatory ginger has an excellent safety profile, and Dr. D almost always recommends it to children and teens with chronic migraines to reduce the frequency of migraine episodes. Dose is one half the adult dose for kids six to twelve of either a ginger-root extract twice a day or a combination ginger/turmeric/bromelain extract once a day. (Remember, long-term use of herbs like ginger and turmeric can promote bleeding to some degree.) For children older than six, Dr. Russ prefers a standardized extract of the herb butterbur, which may be effective against both migraines and allergies. To avoid pyrrolizidine alkaloids that can damage the liver, only use products labeled "PA-free." The typical dose for children under ten years is 25 mg twice daily; older children may need 50 mg twice daily.

▶ Consider a supplement. The vitamin-like compound Coenzyme Q10 (CoQ10) reportedly helps some children with migraines at a dose of 1 mg per pound of body weight a day. CoQ10 is available in liquid form and is easy to administer to children, but it can be costly.

▶ *Massage with herbal oils*. Try massaging the head, neck, and shoulders with a few ounces of olive or almond oil with 1 or 2 drops of either peppermint or arnica essential oil mixed in. Encourage slow, deep breathing during the massage. Be careful not to get essential oils onto the mucous membranes of the nose or mouth.

▶ *Try caffeine*. Paradoxically, the caffeine in a flat cola drink or a cup of green tea can sometimes abort a migraine attack, but this only works in children who do not normally drink caffeinated beverages. In fact, too many caffeinated beverages can trigger migraine.

more on . . .

SERIOUS HEADACHES

Call your doctor or head for the emergency department if your child experiences headaches that:

- ▶ Awaken her from sleep and are relieved by vomiting
- ▶ Cause frequent school absence or recur several times a month
- ▶ Are accompanied by fever and a stiff neck
- ▶ Cause double vision or visual-field problems.
- ▶ Follow a head injury
- ▶ Accompany other neurological signs like new-onset clumsiness

CHAPTER 20

Allergies and Asthma

Allergy-related disease (atopy) has always been a mainstay of our practices. Children come to us with sneezing, wheezing, congestion, runny noses, itchy eyes, chronic cough, bee stings, rashes, gastrointestinal upsets, eczema, recurrent ear or sinus infections, behavioral disorders, and even life-threatening anaphylactic shock. In recent years, however, we've noticed an alarming increase in the number of patients coming through our doors with these complaints.

While it is well known that genetics plays a significant role in the development of allergy and asthma, clearly something more than genes is responsible for the rapid increase in the incidence of these disorders. Genetic changes significant enough to cause this meteoric rise just do not occur on such a broad scale and over so short a period of time. So the question remains: What's causing this epidemic of atopic disease?

Air quality is, not surprisingly, an issue. Higher levels of nitrogen dioxide, sulfur dioxide, particulate matter, and ozone each contribute to an increase in childhood wheezing and emergency department visits for asthma. And it's not just the air outdoors that's at fault. As we've pointed out repeatedly, children today are less active than in previous generations. They spend their days in enclosed schoolrooms, and once home they are fixed to the television or computer, often in rooms with poor ventilation. Such prolonged indoor inactivity exposes them to high levels of indoor allergens, such as dust mites, animal dander, cockroaches, and cigarette smoke.

While these various indoor and outdoor allergens can trigger the onset of symptoms, they don't actually cause the allergy or asthma. Theories abound, but no one knows for certain just what does cause asthma. We lean toward the "hygiene hypothesis" that immune response is altered when our children have less exposure to everyday germs and allergens. More and more studies suggest that infants who are exposed to the great outdoors and all its "dirt," to a dog or cat early in life, or to the common mild childhood infections picked up at day care centers or from older siblings have a smaller incidence of asthma and allergy than those who have less exposure. We think it's quite possible that in our well-intentioned efforts to protect them from germs, we Americans may be doing our children more harm than good. Our overuse of antibiotics also may leave children's immune systems in an unfit, "unexercised" state and make them more susceptible to allergy and asthma. Although the jury is still out on the hygiene hypothesis, wouldn't it be ironic if it turned out that getting dirty in the park as a toddler or playing with a friend with a runny nose actually helped prevent asthma and allergies later?

more on . . .

THE ALLERGIC REACTION

Typically, our protective immune cells recognize an "intruder" and remove it without notice. Sometimes, however, the immune system overreacts to an otherwise harmless particle. We call this an allergic reaction. Cells release chemicals that cause localized or widespread inflammatory changes in the lungs, the gastrointestinal tract, the skin, and other body systems. The resulting symptoms can be mild or severe, ranging from a bothersome swollen lip or runny nose, to the sudden onset of hives (itchy skin wheals or bumps) or wheezing, to the life-threatening anaphylactic reaction, when a person's airways start to swell shut and blood pressure drops precipitously. People who have severe allergic responses, or who have experienced anaphylaxis, are usually prescribed medication such as an EpiPen (or EpiPen Jr. for younger children) that can be self-administered in the earliest stages of an allergic reaction to forestall a more serious attack.

Lessening Allergic Responsiveness

You might be asking yourself how you can prevent your child from developing allergies or asthma when medical science hasn't even determined their cause. But there are a few things we do know that you can do during pregnancy and the first few years of life to lessen the risk of your child developing allergy:

- *Breast-feed for the first four to six months of life.* Despite a few contradictory studies, we recommend breast-feeding as part of a multidisciplinary approach to minimize allergies. Breast-feeding mothers may also be able to reduce their children's sensitization to common allergens even further by limiting their own intake of cow's milk and saturated fats and increasing their intake of omega-3 fatty acids.
- *Introduce new foods slowly.* Once a formula-fed baby is four to six months old or a breast-fed baby is six to seven months old, new foods should be introduced one at a time three or four days apart in order to more easily identify which foods might be problematic. Introducing certain foods before a child's immune system is properly up and running can lead to a higher incidence of allergy, so wait until a child is at least a year old before offering potentially allergenic foods such as liquid cow's milk, whole eggs, peanuts, dark berries, chocolate, shellfish, and exotic fruits like mangoes. In families with peanut allergies, hold off on peanuts or peanut butter until a child is at least three.
- *Do not smoke in the house.* Infant exposure to secondhand smoke is strongly associated with an increased incidence of asthma (as well as sudden infant death syndrome).
- *Try probiotics.* Numerous studies suggest that the incidence of certain allergic disorders can be cut dramatically if expectant moms take probiotics during the last few months of their pregnancy, and if their newborns are then given probiotics for a period of months thereafter.
- *Expose your six-month-old to other children, especially older children.* Experiencing the common, mild infections of childhood early in life may help prevent the subsequent development of allergic disease.

In the following pages we discuss three of the most common childhood allergic disorders: food allergies, allergic rhinitis, and asthma (a fourth, eczema, is discussed in chapter 21). While we have divided these conditions into separate categories, it is important to realize that they overlap and are interrelated. A person with asthma is likely to experience hay fever; a person with food allergies has a high likelihood of having hay fever; certain foods may bring on an episode of asthma, etc. We start with food allergies, however, because the treatment for them is so clear—identify and avoid the offending food.

Food Issues

Food Allergies

Food allergies in children under five are rapidly increasing, as are the numbers of children with multiple food allergies. Peanut allergies alone doubled between 1997 and 2002, which is why some schools now have peanut-free zones in lunchrooms, parents have to be careful what's in the treats for birthday parties, and we all get pretzels instead of peanuts when we fly.

Parents often confuse true food allergies with food sensitivities or intolerances. A true food allergy causes a significant immune reaction. The immune system sees a specific compound in a particular food as a foreign invader and mounts a response that causes such symptoms as bloating, nausea, diarrhea, vomiting, wheezing, flushing, and skin rashes, and may even lead to fatal anaphylaxis. Food allergies are most common during the first two years of life, perhaps because of relatively immature immune and gastrointestinal systems, and are often outgrown.

The foods most commonly implicated in childhood food allergies include cow's milk, wheat, eggs, nuts, corn, shellfish, and soy foods. Children tend to outgrow allergies to milk and egg, but they tend to retain allergies to nuts and shellfish as adults. Adverse reactions (either allergies or sensitivities) to food additives like monosodium glutamate (MSG), tartrazine (FD&C Yellow No. 5), benzoic acid, and sulfites are also common during childhood.

Skin or blood (RAST) testing performed by a physician can identify substances to which your child is allergic. Your child may have to avoid certain foods entirely, as increased exposure to the food can increase the severity of the reaction to it. Children with serious food allergies should carry preventive medications in case of life-threatening anaphylactic reactions. To protect your child—and his friends—you will have to become a careful reader of food and vitamin labels to make sure a potential allergen is not lurking far down the ingredient list. There are books and Internet sites listed in the resource section that can help you.

Food Sensitivities and Intolerances

Food sensitivities and intolerances are real and problematic, but they are not true allergies. Your child may have an intolerance or sensitivity if there are certain foods that just don't "sit right" with her stomach, or if she feels tired or "heavy" a few hours after eating certain foods.

Food sensitivity may actually cause some of the same symptoms as food allergy, but a different immune mechanism is at work. Sometimes these mild-to-moderate inflammatory reactions may be delayed as much as 12 to 48 hours, making diagnosis more difficult. Common triggers for food sensitivities are milk, wheat, corn, aged cheese, and food additives. Food sensitivities may be expressed as digestive difficulties, joint pain, rash, a severe case of cradle cap, fatigue, difficulty concentrating, recurrent respiratory tract infections, nasal congestion, or breathing problems. Some experts believe that food sensitivities play a role in the development of recurrent ear infections, headaches, behavioral problems like attention deficit disorder, and even chronic diseases like rheumatoid arthritis.

Food intolerance is not an immune problem but a digestive problem that arises when a child lacks the proper enzyme to break down a particular food in the gut. For instance, a child who is lactose intolerant lacks enough of the enzyme lactase to break down milk sugar (lactose). Common trouble foods are dairy foods, wheat, and the sweeteners fructose and sorbitol. People who are intolerant to a certain food may still be able to eat it if they supplement with the missing enzyme, or eat the food less often or in smaller amounts.

Tools for Dealing with Food Intolerance and Sensitivity

If you believe a food sensitivity or intolerance is making your child uncomfortable or even sick, you can help your child's doctor uncover the culprit using two powerful tools: the food diary and the elimination diet.

- *In the food diary you record every food your child eats each day, and any changes you see in his physical, mental, or emotional state.* Use the diary to look for patterns, and try to pinpoint problem foods.

- *An elimination diet, or food challenge, is designed to identify foods that may be causing symptoms.* The easiest way to do an elimination diet is to pick a food to which your child is most likely to be sensitive, like dairy or eggs, and then eliminate it completely from his diet for two weeks. Notice how he is feeling and acting at that time, and document symptoms in the daily diary. At the end of the trial, gently reintroduce the food into his diet. If there is a significant change, such as bloating, congestion, or headaches, he may indeed be sensitive to that particular food.

If your child is found to be sensitive to or intolerant of a certain food, it does not mean that she cannot ever eat that food. She may just need to eat it in smaller amounts or less often, or avoid it just before a big trip. One way to minimize the chances of developing a food allergy or sensitivity is to vary your child's diet as much as possible.

more on . . .

FOOD TESTING

We have seen a number of people who were advised not to eat a broad array of foods, including some of the foods they enjoyed most, after blood tests reportedly revealed possible food sensitivities. We see no reason to avoid a favorite food solely because of a test result if your child hasn't experienced any unpleasant symptoms when eating the food. By the same token, if your child continues to experience adverse reactions to a food that did not show up as allergenic in testing, trust the evidence of your eyes and limit the food.

Asthma and Allergic Rhinitis

Asthma and allergic rhinitis are best seen as variations on a single disease process, with one affecting the lower airways (lungs) and the other affecting the upper airways (nose). While the conventional approach is to cover up the symptoms associated with these disorders, the integrative pediatrician takes aim at their cause as well.

None of the following recommendations is a substitute for conventional medical therapy, but individually or in combination these five strategies may help your child experience allergic or asthmatic symptoms less often, with greater ease and greater sense of control over the situation, and they may enable your doctor to minimize medications previously felt necessary. The treatment of any childhood illness is successful only when there is a partnership among the child, the parent, and the physician, and this is especially true in the treatment of allergic conditions.

Reducing Allergic Response

1. *Stop smoking*. Exposure to passive tobacco smoke worsens coughing and wheezing and makes children more susceptible to viral respiratory tract infections.

2. *Serve more fruits and vegetables*. The high antioxidant content of a diet rich in fruits and vegetables might minimize susceptibility to irritants and allergens. Organic produce reduces exposure to potentially allergenic agricultural chemicals. It's best if your children get their antioxidants through proper eating, but if that isn't possible, a few studies do suggest that supplementation with a standardized extract of French maritime pine bark (*Pinus pinaster*) called Pycnogenol may be useful.

3. *Serve foods containing anti-inflammatory fats and oils*. Since allergy and asthma are primarily inflammatory disorders, eating foods that contain high levels of anti-inflammatory omega-3 fatty acids such as salmon, sardines, walnuts, and ground flaxseeds could prove helpful. If your kids won't eat those foods, consider a daily supplement of pure fish oil. Limit

pro-inflammatory polyunsaturated and partially hydrogenated oils and also foods cooked in them.

4. *Keep an eye on dairy products*. Some components of milk may increase inflammation and mucus secretion. It is worthwhile to give your child a trial period free of dairy products to see if this improves the condition. (If you do, provide enough calcium from other sources to meet daily requirements.)

5. *Consider probiotics*. A probiotic supplement may decrease activity of IgE, the antibody most closely associated with allergic reactions, and also prevent allergens from moving beyond the gastrointestinal tract.

6. *Reduce exposure to potential environmental triggers*. This includes such factors as pollen, molds, dust-mite or cockroach waste, and air pollution. More detailed suggestions on how to do this appear later in this chapter.

Allergic Rhinitis

Allergic rhinitis (an allergic inflammation of the mucous membranes of the nose) is the single most common chronic disease of childhood. You may well be familiar with the symptoms of *seasonal allergic rhinitis* (more commonly called "hay fever") with its coughing, sneezing, congested nose, and watery, itchy eyes. These symptoms rise and fall with the appearance of various plant and tree pollens, with spring and summer being the worst times of the year for many people. In contrast, the similar symptoms of *perennial allergic rhinitis* occur year-round, mostly because of chronic exposure to animal dander, dust mites, or the airborne spores of mold. Allergic rhinitis may also be an unrecognized factor in recurrent sinus and ear infections, sleep disorders, postnasal drip, chronic cough, mouth breathing, eye blinking, fatigue, and difficulties in concentration.

In addition to the general suggestions above, we recommend seven actions to take against allergic rhinitis to help reduce your child's exposure to triggers, relieve symptoms, and decrease reliance on over-the-counter or prescription drugs.

Dealing with Allergic Rhinitis

1. *Clean off pollen.* Have your child shower or bathe at night or after playing outside to get pollen off skin and hair.

2. *Reduce exposure to other allergens.* Take precautions against dust mites and cockroaches (see page 274). The new UVC vacuum cleaners that use a germicidal form of ultraviolet light look very promising for controlling dust mites. Keep humidity in the house low to discourage molds and mites. Keep pets outdoors if possible, and definitely out of your child's bedroom.

3. *Take off your shoes at the door.* That way fewer pollens are tracked into the house.

4. *Filter the air.* Watch the news for pollen counts, and keep your child indoors with the windows closed when counts are high. Consider adding a HEPA (high efficiency particulate air) filter to central ductwork to clean the air indoors during the season, and change the filters often. Clean the house frequently with a vacuum fitted with a HEPA filter.

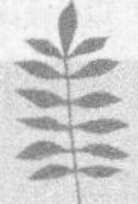

TIP: Don't use an ozone generator to clean the air. These machines could make asthma worse by increasing air levels of toxic ozone gas.

5. *Give more liquids.* Mucous membranes that are appropriately moist are able to perform their immune functions more competently.

6. *Try a homeopathic remedy.* Over-the-counter single homeopathic remedies aimed only at relieving symptoms, such as *Allium* for runny nose and *Euphrasia* for itchy eyes, may be helpful.

7. *Try a botanical remedy.* The herb butterbur (*Petasites hybridus*) has been shown in some studies to work as well as prescription drugs and may have the added benefit of helping to prevent asthma attacks and migraines too.

Medications for Allergic Rhinitis

If these natural approaches don't give your child enough relief during peak season, your child's doctor may suggest a prescription drug to try to control symptoms. Among the most common:

- *Leukotriene inhibitors.* A drug like montelukast (Singulair) is safe and effective for allergic rhinitis and can be used for up to six months at a time with very few side effects.

- *Antihistamines.* Antihistamines short-circuit the biochemical histamine reaction that causes most of the symptoms of an allergic response. Older varieties of antihistamine, such as diphenhydramine (Benadryl) and especially hydroxyzine (Atarax), produce significant side effects including either sedation or hyperactivity, impaired learning in children, and drying of the mucous membranes. The newer prescription and over-the-counter antihistamines like loratadine (Claritin), fexofenadine (Allegra), and cetirizine hydrochloride (Zyrtec) have a better side-effect profile, although Dr. D has seen several patients develop incontinence on Claritin that resolved only when the medication was stopped.

- *Decongestants.* Though they are approved for children over six, we strongly recommend against the use of over-the-counter medications like pseudoephedrine (Sudafed). They have very little benefit and commonly cause side effects like insomnia and agitation when they are taken orally.

- *Immunotherapy.* Allergy shots continued for months or years can eradicate hay fever—though this is not a popular therapy with children.

- *Steroids.* Although steroid nasal sprays can be very effective against the symptoms of allergic rhinitis, they suppress immune response. We do prescribe short courses of steroids for severe situations or when a child has not responded to conventional medications. We try to use the least potent steroid at the smallest possible dosage that obtains a beneficial effect. In our experience, the corticosteroid mometasone furoate monohydrate (Nasonex) is the safest for children and has little effect on immune response.

Asthma

Until recently, asthma was considered to be a problem caused by the constriction of overly reactive airways. Asthma is now defined as a chronic inflammatory condition of the lower airways that leads to recurrent reversible bronchospasm. The airways narrow when the muscles of the breathing tube contract and when swelling, mucus, and cellular debris build up in response to an inflammatory stimulus. If not recognized early and treated adequately, recurrent inflammation can cause long-term changes within the airways that lead to impaired lung function in adulthood. But diagnosing asthma in an infant or toddler can prove to be very tricky.

Not all children who wheeze have asthma. In fact, most do not. Most children will outgrow this tendency toward reactive airways after the toddler years. Children who have families with a history of wheezing in adulthood are more likely to develop asthma that they will not outgrow.

Asthma can be divided into two broad categories: allergic and nonallergic. Allergic asthma is triggered by many of the same things that initiate hay fever. Nonallergic asthma is most often triggered by cold or polluted air, vigorous play or exercise, emotional upset, or upper respiratory infection. (Most children who develop airway obstruction in response to a viral infection do grow out of the condition.) While we separate the two classes of asthma, almost all children have some component of allergy to their asthma that causes their lungs to react as they do.

The symptoms of an asthma episode—wheezing, shortness of breath, tightness in the chest, a laugh that turns into a cough—can be quite frightening to both child and parent. If the episode is a severe one, a child's nostrils may flare, the muscles between her ribs may retract during inhalation, and she may not be moving enough air to even produce a wheeze. In the worst of situations, the airways are so closed off that the child turns blue and ultimately becomes so tired from the effort of breathing that she stops breathing on her own. Every year hundreds of children die from asthma, despite all the drugs available to treat the condition. Is it any wonder we take asthma seriously?

Any child who wheezes regularly should see a doctor for evaluation. Currently, conventional asthma treatment for the 5 million children with asthma in this country rests on two prescription drugs, a daily one for prevention of attacks and another one that is used as needed to treat attacks. However, we have both successfully treated children with asthma with minimal use of the usual prescription drugs. Our individualized integrative asthma programs focus on giving children and their parents the tools to prevent or control asthma episodes with both natural approaches and, as necessary, prescription medications.

Dealing with Asthma

1. *Follow our general allergy program above*. Be especially careful to feed your child a healthy diet, as asthma has been linked to a lack of fresh fruits and vegetables, low intake of omega-3 fatty acids, and an excess of processed and fast foods that can increase inflammation. Treat allergic rhinitis, which can trigger asthma episodes.

2. *Make your child a partner in his asthma program*. To avoid frequent trips to the emergency department or long-standing problems in adulthood, your child must take her medication as directed. The best way to instill compliance is to make sure your child understands the importance of the various elements in her treatment program, and give her some sense of control over the program.

Your child's doctor or nurse should:

- Make sure both you and your child understand the process at work in asthma.
- Reinforce oral instructions for prevention and treatment of asthma episodes with written materials.
- Teach you both the proper use of an *inhaler*—a device that distributes asthma medication into the airways—so the medication doesn't end up sprayed onto the back of the throat instead of into the lungs.
- Teach younger children proper use of a *spacer* attached to the inhaler.
- Teach you both how to use a device called a *peak-flow meter* if your child's respiratory function is to be monitored at home,

and the *home nebulizer*, a clever device that aerosolizes medications that open airways (usually albuterol or levalbuterol), if one is prescribed. The nebulizer can deliver both preventive and acute-care medicines for asthma, and cut back on visits to the doctor or the emergency department.

3. *Reduce exposure to dust mites and cockroaches.* Though we can't see them, microscopic insects called dust mites live on and all around us, eating dead skin. Many asthmatic children are allergic to these mites and their waste products. To limit your child's exposure to dust mites—especially in the bedroom, where they are most often found—remove carpeting and curtains, or vacuum frequently with a UVC vacuum cleaner with a HEPA filter and wash sheets and stuffed toys in hot water every week. Cockroaches and their feces are another trigger for asthma, so don't leave food around to attract them, and wash floors and counters frequently to eliminate their debris.

4. *Provide training in a mind/body technique.* Stress can bring on or worsen an episode of asthma, and relaxation techniques can improve the efficiency of breathing as well as the perception of changes within the lungs. Other techniques, such as massage therapy, have been shown beneficial for young children with asthma, and yoga practice has likewise resulted in a reduction in stress, an enhanced sense of well-being, improved results on some tests of breathing function, and in some cases a reduced need for medication. Even the simple activity of keeping a journal may help older children minimize systemic inflammation associated with asthma. Such techniques may be useful for parents too, so children don't "catch" their anxiety.

5. *Get rid of mold.* Find and repair leaks and other sources of excess moisture in the house. Use a dehumidifier in damp rooms like basements, and remove any mold that collects in showers, sinks, and garbage cans.

6. *Keep pets out of the bedroom, and if possible, out of the house.* This is a tough one, but while exposure to pets early in infancy may be protective,

their dander may be a trigger for older kids with existing asthma. Wash your pets at least once a week.

7. *Partner with your child's teacher*. Many schoolrooms contain triggers such as mold, pets, or plants that can induce reactions in children. Make certain the teacher understands your child's condition, and the need to keep an inhaler on hand (not in the nurse's office) in case of difficulty.

8. *Maintain healthy body weight*. Obesity doubles the risk of new-onset asthma in children.

9. *Try a supplement*. Mushroom or astragalus tonics may boost the immune system and help prevent upper respiratory tract infections that lead to wheezing. Botanical extracts of butterbur or French maritime pine bark may offer some protection from severe asthma attacks. Long-term oral magnesium supplementation may help open up airways, but be sure to talk with your child's doctor first, as too much magnesium can be dangerous.

10. *Sign up for flu shots*. If your child has asthma, be sure she gets an annual flu shot. The pneumonia shot (Prevnar) may be helpful as well.

11. *Rule out reflux*. "Silent" GERD has been associated with asthma. Have your child evaluated for reflux if his condition is not responding to treatment.

12. *Promote vigorous play*. People who exercise on a regular basis show a decrease in frequency of asthma episodes, a reduced need for medication, and an increased sense of well-being and self-confidence. Exercise can *trigger* symptoms in some kids with nonallergic asthma, who may need to take a hit of the inhaler five or ten minutes before engaging in physical activity.

13. *Give Chinese medicine a try*. Dr. Russ has seen the conditions of a number of patients with asthma improve significantly after acupuncture and/or Chinese herbs. (See chapter 13.)

14. *Try manual medicine*. An osteopath, a well-trained massage therapist, and some chiropractors can work on the muscles surrounding the chest wall to allow more efficient movement of the rib cage, which may translate into more efficient air exchange.

15. *Make sure your child drinks enough water*. It is especially important to keep your child drinking frequent sips of water during asthma flares, as she can easily become dehydrated while working so hard at breathing.

Prescription Medications for Asthma

There is an array of prescription drugs available to help children with asthma. When medication is necessary we usually prescribe regular preventive use of a leukotriene inhibitor or inhaled steroid drug to minimize the inflammation that can trigger an episode of asthma. We also prescribe drugs called beta agonists to be used when needed to relax the airways during an acute asthma attack. These drugs can be quite beneficial, but they may have significant side effects, so our goal is to use them at the lowest possible dosage and frequency that gives a child the desired improvement.

- *Leukotriene inhibitors*. This class of drugs—such as montelukast (Singulair)—inhibit the production of inflammatory mediators of allergy and asthma. They are good for long-term use to prevent asthma episodes. They can be used in children as young as six months, have a great safety profile, cause few side effects, and are easily delivered to children as granules sprinkled on food.

- *Steroids*. Anti-inflammatory steroids are very effective at reducing inflammation, and the newer inhaled steroids like budesonide (Pulmicort) have good safety profiles in children. Oral steroids should be reserved only for severe exacerbations as more chronic use of them suppresses adrenal function and can cause mood disturbances, delayed growth, and loss of calcium from bones.

- *Inhaled beta agonists*. The mainstay of treatment for acute asthma, most of these medications quickly relax and open up the airways. (The exception, a beta agonist called salmeterol, is actually a preventive and is not used for acute situations.) Both short-acting and long-acting forms are available but concerns have arisen regarding the safety of long-acting agents. Be sure to speak with your doctor about issues related to both safety and effectiveness if a long-acting beta agonist is recommended for your child. If your child has to use short-acting inhaled beta agonists frequently, you should pay more attention to adequately controlling the condition with preventive drugs and natural measures.

CHAPTER 21

Skin Problems

Is there anything that feels softer and smells better than a baby's neck? Yet the very perfection and innocence of a baby's skin signal its vulnerability. Skin problems like prickly heat and diaper rash vex babies, and as they grow, other signs of trouble are likely to show on their skin as well. These symptoms may be caused by systemic problems like chicken pox or food allergy, or by conditions more specific to the skin, such as ringworm or cradle cap. In this chapter we describe an integrative pediatric approach to eight common skin conditions of childhood.

But first, a little about the care and feeding of baby skin. Babies are born with a protective waxy coating called the vernix over their immature skin. As they make the adjustment to an air environment after all that time floating in amniotic fluid, their skin may peel. Don't rush to apply creams and lotions, as this is a natural process. Don't use soap on infants under six months, either, as soaps dissolve grease and oil. The skin's thin layer of natural oils is the best protection a newborn has to keep germs out and fluids in while the skin is slowly building its immune defenses.

After the age of six months, it's fine to use a mild nondrying soap or cleanser with the bath. When choosing soap or any product applied to baby's skin, look for one with the shortest list of chemical additives. Many of these cosmetic products—

even some of the ones meant for babies—contain fragrances and other chemicals that, while not a problem for adults, may irritate baby's more permeable skin. (See Resources.)

Cradle Cap

Infantile seborrheic dermatitis (cradle cap) is a common condition in newborns. It's a malfunction of the young sebaceous (oil) glands in the middle layer of the skin that causes flakes of skin to be welded together by excess oil into thick, yellowish scales. Cradle cap looks like an industrial-sized case of dandruff, but it doesn't bother baby and will eventually go away on its own. You can speed healing along by massaging your baby's head gently with a little room-temperature extra-virgin olive oil two or three times a week. The olive oil will moisturize the skin and loosen scalp scales. Breast-feeding moms can add more ground flaxseed and cold-water fish (or fish oil supplements) to their diet to enrich their milk with more anti-inflammatory compounds. Severe cradle cap can also be a sign of allergy to milk or other foods. Try eliminating possible triggers from a nursing mom's diet, or switch bottle-fed babies to a predigested formula.

Prickly Heat

A baby's automatic heating and cooling system is a work in progress for its first few months of life, so they overheat easily. Their sweat ducts are immature, so sweat gets trapped under the skin and can cause a red, itchy rash known as *prickly heat* (miliaria). While the rash usually occurs on the face, it may also occur on the body, especially if a baby has been heavily swaddled.

You can prevent prickly heat by dressing your baby in layers easily adjustable to changes in temperature, by avoiding the use of heavy, oil-based skin creams, and by leaning more toward cotton and other breathable fibers.

You can treat prickly heat by cooling your child down with a lukewarm (not cold) bath and a change to lighter-weight clothing. To prevent scratching and possible skin infections, ease the itching with cold compresses or by adding colloidal oatmeal bath products or plain old baking soda to the bath. A light application of baby cornstarch or anti-inflammatory calendula lotion afterward might also be helpful.

Diaper Rash

Most parents are familiar with the irritation and redness that will at some time or another appear in the diaper area. Diaper rash can be caused by a number of different factors, including prolonged contact with urine or stool, excess heat and humidity caused by restricted air circulation, friction, fungal infection, and allergic reaction to diapers, lotions, wipes, or even the detergents used to launder cloth diapers.

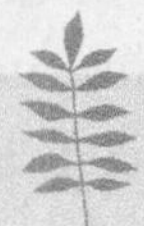

TIP: Breast-fed babies get less diaper rash, apparently because their stool is less alkaline.

Preventing Diaper Rash

- *Change diapers frequently*. This reduces the length of time a child's skin is exposed to urine and stool. Very young babies need to have their diapers changed eight to ten times a day.

- *Experiment to see whether your baby's skin does better with cloth or disposable diapers*. If you choose disposables, look for styles or brands that are soft enough and fit well enough not to cause friction and that don't contain any materials that cause skin reaction in your baby.

- *Avoid tight-fitting diapers and plastic pants*. You want air to circulate in there. Watch for new breathable disposables, and limit the amount of time your child wears plastic pants.

- *Don't use wipes or other bottom cleaners that contain alcohol, fragrance, or other chemicals that can be irritating*. Just use a cotton washcloth or soft gauze and warm water to wash the diaper area, and be sure to dry thoroughly.

- *Don't overdo baby powders*. Try not to spread the powder all around or near baby's face, as inhalation of powders or talc can cause respiratory problems in babies (and adults). Cornstarch-based powders may be less problematic.

Treating Diaper Rash

▸ *Give baby's bottom an airing.* Put your child down for a nap without a diaper on a waterproof sheet or let her bottom have some time out in the fresh warm air.

▸ *Apply a thick layer of a barrier cream every time you change your baby's diaper until diaper rash is healed.* Wash baby's bottom gently with lukewarm water only, and slather on a cream or ointment that contains zinc oxide and a gentle moisturizer. Next time you clean baby's bottom, try to leave a thin layer of the cream on as scrubbing it all away can slough off new skin. This is especially important if a baby has persistent diarrhea that has burned the upper layers of skin and left some of the skin in the area raw. Some parents prefer to apply egg white, or a blend of oatmeal, and either flax or olive oil intermittently, and these natural methods work fine too, especially for older children.

▸ *Consider dietary factors.* If a child's bottom becomes raw after each bowel movement, you should also consider potential allergens like milk, which can make stool acidic enough to burn little tushies. Eliminate new foods that raise your suspicions and see if the problem clears up.

TIP: Use over-the-counter ointments that contain corticosteroids for diaper rash only when prescribed by your baby's doctor. These drugs are more easily absorbed in infants, who may therefore be more vulnerable to their negative side effects.

Take your child to the doctor if diaper rash persists or worsens, because he may have a fungal or bacterial skin infection. Most commonly, the cause is an overgrowth of *Candida*, a yeast that typically lives on the human body in harmony with other organisms. Sometimes changes in the usual environment, such as increased dampness or alkalinity, upset the normal balance of skin flora, and excessive *Candida* growth will cause a bumpy red rash, usually concentrated in the skin folds and sometimes accompanied by peeling. There may be additional red bumps at a distance from the main rash (satellite lesions), and perhaps a yeast infection called *thrush* in the mouth as well.

Typical treatment for yeast is a light application of an over-the-counter or prescription antifungal cream such as clotrimazole or nystatin. More potent antifungal skin creams are also available and highly effective, but we think they carry unnecessary risks to a young child. We don't usually recommend oral antifungals for diaper candidiasis. We often supplement antifungal therapy with a probiotic, either for the mother if the child is breast-fed or for the child herself, to maintain beneficial flora in the intestinal tract, mouth, and other areas lined with mucous membranes.

Bacterial infections of the diaper area are also common, typically showing oozing and blisters. A swab culture will identify the culprit and allow your child's doctor to prescribe the proper antibiotic.

Atopic Dermatitis/Eczema

Atopic dermatitis, often called *eczema,* is an increasingly common inflammatory condition of both infants and children frequently accompanied by allergic rhinitis or asthma. About 10 percent of children suffer from this skin condition, a percentage that has mysteriously doubled since the 1950s and 1960s. Fortunately, many children with atopic dermatitis outgrow it by their teens.

The hallmark of this chronic condition is severe itching and inflammation that eventually results in blisters, scales, and other lesions on the skin, especially of the face and the folds of the elbows and knees. There is some degree of inherited susceptibility involved, but atopic dermatitis appears to be driven mostly by environmental factors such as diet, chemical irritants, and stress.

An integrative program for atopic dermatitis encompasses our general program for reducing severity and frequency of inflammation found in previous chapters as well as the following specific suggestions:

- *Look for food allergens*. Breast-feeding moms should eliminate potential allergens such as nuts and dairy. Bottle-fed babies should be getting a formula fortified with omega-3 fatty acids or switched to a hypoallergenic formula to reduce possible sensitization to dairy. Consider a food trial and challenge for older children.

▶ *Look for and deal with environmental irritants in the home or day care center.*

▶ *Protect natural defenses*. It appears that the skin's ability to act as a barrier is compromised in kids with atopic dermatitis, so you want to do what you can to help it hold water. Hot baths dissolve away natural skin oils, so bathe or shower children briefly every day in warm water. When they're dirty, use a mild soap based on oatmeal, aloe, or calendula. Don't use bubble bath, which contains a lot of chemicals, and be sure to shampoo hair at the end of a bath so the child doesn't linger in shampoo.

▶ *Use a moisturizer*. Find one with as few synthetic ingredients as possible and use it immediately after bathing to seal in moisture. Reapply several times a day. Don't use lotions, creams, or other toiletries that contain alcohol, which is very drying to the skin.

▶ *Dress your child in soft, breathable natural fabrics as much as possible.* Cotton clothing is ideal.

▶ *Ease itchy skin with a handful of oatmeal or baking soda in the bath*. Rinse the child in clean water afterward. You can also soothe the itch with warm tea bag compresses of chamomile or a moisturizing oatmeal pack. Do not apply these compresses to open, weeping skin because of the risk of infection.

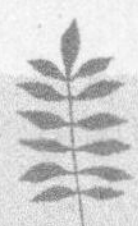

TIP: To make an oatmeal pack, mix oatmeal and distilled water in a blender to a paste-like consistency, add a tablespoon or so of flax or olive oil, blend again, and apply.

▶ *Put cotton socks on your child's hands at night*. This will decrease the risk of infection from itches scratched.

▶ *Increase your child's intake of essential fatty acids through ground flaxseed or supplemental fish oils*.

▶ *Try calendula skin cream.* This herbal remedy both soothes the skin and reduces inflammation. Pure aloe vera gel may also be soothing. Don't use on broken skin.

▶ *Switch laundry soaps, or run clothes through two rinses.* Sensitivity to ingredients in popular detergents is not uncommon, even in those with babies pictured on the package.

▶ *Consider probiotics.* Research suggests that probiotic supplementation during the last few weeks of pregnancy and the first few months of the newborn's life can halve the incidence of eczema in families with a history of allergic disorders. Breast-feeding moms can supplement with fish oils and probiotic products containing lactobacilli or bifidobacteria. Older kids can also take the supplements, or small amounts of the probiotic can be added to formula or food. Both moms and kids can eat yogurt with active bacteria.

▶ *Practice mind/body techniques.* These help manage stress and should be a mainstay of treatment in kids older than five or six. Consider guided imagery, self-hypnosis, and/or biofeedback for treatment as well.

If itching and scaling worsens, we might consider using a low-potency (1 percent hydrocortisone or less) cortisone cream with limits on the amount and duration of treatment. We are very cautious with these admittedly useful drugs, because their side effects can be serious, especially in babies. The armpits, groin, and face are particularly absorbent areas of the skin on an infant, so steroid creams should never be applied in those places unless your doctor has ordered it (and even then, use them minimally and cautiously).

Sometimes a severe case of atopic dermatitis may require treatment with antibiotics if repeated scratching leads to infection by *Staphylococcus aureus* or other bacteria. If the typical red, scaly, oozing rash of eczema becomes fiery red or develops pustules, bring your child to the doctor to see if an antibiotic is necessary.

Hives

Hives (urticaria) are a pretty common allergic reaction in children. These fast-rising, usually itchy, patches (or wheals) occur in response to stress, a bacterial or viral infection, or an allergenic food, chemical, or drug. Hives often resolve without their cause ever being known, but they may persist for weeks. Once a raging case of hives gets going, it may take two to three weeks to cool it down, as the immune system must go through its full cycle of response to the offending agent.

A mild antihistamine like Benadryl (sedating) or Zyrtec (nonsedating) or oral steroids may be prescribed to control symptoms. Older kids may benefit from mind/body therapies, especially hypnosis, or from supplements such as quercetin or butterbur. *Take your child to the doctor* for an allergy workup if hives are persistent. *Take your child to the emergency department* if hives are accompanied by any signs of respiratory distress.

Ringworm

Ringworm (tinea) actually has nothing to do with worms, but is a fungal infection that typically strikes children on the scalp or the body. It starts as a small scaly spot, which enlarges to form a ring with raised red edges with a clearing in the middle. When it occurs on the scalp, hair within the ring breaks off or falls out, leaving a bald spot. It may be itchy.

Ringworm on the body can be cured by application of 1½ tablespoons of 5 to 10 percent tea tree oil diluted in a cup of warm water three or four times a day for two weeks, or by application of over-the-counter antifungal creams such as Lotrimin. Ringworm on the scalp can be cured only by a prescription oral antifungal drug. Your child's doctor will probably monitor liver function, which oral antifungal drugs can temporarily impair. A shampoo containing selenium sulfide may also be recommended to kill the fungus. Hair loss from scalp ringworm can become permanent if the infection is not treated appropriately. The condition is very contagious, which is why children should be taught never to share combs, barrettes, scrunchies, hats, or pillows.

Head Lice

These tiny bloodsucking insects can cause great embarrassment the first time your child's school or day care center calls to ask you to come pick up your child because she has head lice. The sight of little nits (louse eggs) that look like rice firmly attached to some of your darling's hairs generally triggers a frenzy of cleaning and disinfection of both child and environment to assuage a shameful sense that child and family are somehow "dirty."

The sense of shame is unwarranted. Head lice don't carry disease, and children of all degrees of cleanliness catch them (as do their parents—another nasty surprise). The usual recommendation for getting rid of head lice is a shampoo containing either a chemical or a natural pesticide. We don't recommend shampoos based on pesticides like lindane or malathion, and we prefer to save plant-based pyrethrin shampoos for stubborn cases that do not resolve with less toxic approaches, because lice appear to be developing resistance to it. We have hopes for a new nontoxic, pesticide-free product just being launched.

Dr. D recommends smothering lice by applying a heavy coating of margarine, mayonnaise, or Vaseline to a child's hair and scalp. Cover with a shower cap or plastic wrap and leave on several hours or overnight before washing it out. It's a messy therapy, but it has shown good results. Dr. Russ prefers a remedy passed on to him by Dr. Andrew Weil: Mix 2 ounces of olive or coconut oil with 20 drops of tea tree oil and 10 drops of either rosemary, lavender, or lemon essential oil and rub it into the scalp and hair. Cover with a towel or shower cap for one hour (no longer). In either case, wash hair thoroughly to remove these oily substances and comb, comb, comb with a fine-toothed nit comb. A handheld magnifying glass can be useful in looking for the pearly nits, which especially like the areas behind the ears and along the nape of the neck. Nits take two weeks to hatch, so do follow-up checks on your child's clean dry hair occasionally throughout that period to reduce the risk of recurrence.

In the meantime, soak combs and brushes your child has used in alcohol for an hour. Put your child's bedding and the stuffed animals he sleeps with in plastic bags for three or four days until nits have hatched and lice have died from lack of food. Follow through with similar procedures in shared resting places in the classroom or day care center.

Molluscum

Molluscum contagiosum (MC) is a long-lasting and contagious "rash" of small, pearly, domed lesions that become soft and indented with time. It's common in children, who haven't yet developed immunity to the virus that causes it. MC is usually found on the face, thighs, underarms, eyelids, or neck, and while unsightly, is not usually itchy. It's spread by contact, so if your child has MC, it is important that they not spread the rash or give it to others by touching or scratching the lesions. Make sure they don't share towels or sports equipment either.

Treat MC by dabbing 1 or 2 drops of undiluted tea tree oil on top of each little wart with a cotton swab every morning for six to eight weeks. You can also cover the individual warts with good old duct tape at night, to prevent scratching.

CHAPTER 22

Problems of Attention

Children are active and full of energy by nature. That's what makes it so tricky to tell the difference between a child who is naturally active and one who is hyperactive. It could be that someone—a teacher, perhaps—has already suggested that the son who always seems to be in motion or the daughter who lives in a dream world may have attention deficit disorder (ADD). So what does ADD mean, does the term really apply to your child, and what do you do if it does?

Various medical, educational, and psychological groups use the terms *ADD* and *ADHD* differently. For purposes of this chapter, we use ADD as an umbrella term covering all three attention disorders—attention deficit without hyperactivity (ADD), attention deficit with hyperactivity (ADHD), and undifferentiated attention deficit. These three neurobehavioral disorders of attention represent a spectrum featuring various degrees of inattention, hyperactivity, and impulsivity. In young boys, ADD appears most often as an inability to sit still, compulsive talking, and impulsive or aggressive behavior. In girls it presents most often as daydreaming, absentmindedness, and difficulty in concentrating. Someone with true ADD has a greater chance of also having depression, anxiety, or a conduct disorder, especially if peer relationships suffer.

A diagnosis of ADD is easiest when impulsivity or hyperactivity accompanies attention problems. Unfortunately, a child with an attention disorder who lacks these two active symptoms may be mistakenly labeled lazy or unintelligent by both school personnel and family members. This is both unfair and unfortunate, as many children with ADD are extremely bright and creative.

Most experts agree that ADD is not simply a behavioral quirk but rather a complex multifactorial disorder of brain chemistry and function influenced by family history, prenatal influences, premature birth, environment, upbringing, and differences in the timing of brain development. Because so many factors influence ADD, signs and symptoms vary and children with similar symptoms may respond to different therapies.

There is a lot of concern about the supposed "epidemic" of ADD in kids today. Prescriptions for the ADD drug Ritalin (methylphenidate) doubled or tripled in the five years from 1991 to 1995 in both children less than five years of age (despite warnings on the label against its use in children under six), and those five to fourteen, and continue to escalate. About 2.5 million American children are currently taking drugs for ADD. Is this astonishing increase proof of an epidemic, evidence of environmental toxicity, a sign of changing societal expectations, or a trend in diagnosis?

Diagnosing Attention Disorders

Unfortunately, there are no laboratory tests that can determine ADD. Medical guidelines for the diagnosis of ADD have varied by specialty, and the diagnosis is often informally made by parents, day care providers, teachers, principals, and other educational professionals. As a result, many kids who do not really have ADD are given drugs for the disorder, and many kids who have less recognizable forms of the problem may not get treatment at all. Often children incorrectly diagnosed with ADD actually have learning disabilities that respond dramatically to individualized educational approaches.

It is important to rule out other causes of restlessness, inattention, and impulsivity before deciding on a diagnosis of ADD. Definitions of what constitutes hyperactivity can be pretty subjective. One teacher's energetic and creative student can be another's irritating interrupter. Children can act out or tune out because they're bored, don't get along with the teacher, have different learning styles, or are too immature for the amount of discipline required. Because of the multifactorial nature of ADD and its possible confusion and coexistence with other conditions, a pediatrician should make this diagnosis only after several visits with the child and discussions with the child's parents, teachers, school counselors, coaches, or other appropriate sources of information concerning the child's behavior at home, in school, or on the playing fields. The diagnosis of ADD requires that a significant number of symptoms be evident at more than one physical location and consistently for at least six months.

Treating Attention Disorders

The treatment plan for kids with ADD should take a multidisciplinary approach that includes educating parents and child, teaching coping and self-regulatory skills, partnering with educators on learning strategies and tools, modifying and structuring the environment, and—in more severe cases—medication. However, too many practitioners are not taking the time to make a reliable diagnosis, and too many families are just being offered the "quick fix" of stimulant drugs. This trend is propelled by school systems that press for stimulant drugs as a form of behavior management. We don't think any parent should seek out medications for their child—especially psychotropic drugs—without the child first going through a rigorous diagnostic process.

more on . . .

OTHER CAUSES OF INATTENTION

Difficulties with schoolwork or behavior can also be caused by a wide range of emotional, social, or medical problems, including hearing or vision impairment, family stress, lead poisoning, thyroid disease, hunger, recurrent ear infections, disturbed sleep, a disorganized home environment, epilepsy, a learning disorder, anemia, pinworms, food allergies or sensitivities, head trauma, overconsumption of caffeinated or sugary beverages, too much media stimulation, or the side effects of certain medications.

The drugs most commonly used for ADHD are central nervous system stimulants, most often Ritalin (methylphenidate) or its longer-acting forms (such as Focalin), although Dexedrine (dextroamphetamine) or Adderal (mixed amphetamine salts) may be prescribed. Though it seems illogical, these central nervous system stimulants actually allow children with ADD to focus and gain some control over their actions—though it may just be a temporary solution. While the drugs appear to improve organizational skills and handwriting, they seem to improve academic accomplishments or social skills only in a small group of kids, most likely those who have a true chemical imbalance. Prescription stimulants should be used only as part of a home and school program that also encompasses behavioral and educational approaches. (Nonstimulant agents, such as atomoxetine, are also available for treatment but are similarly plagued by significant side effects.)

We have three big issues with the routine prescription of prescription stimulants to children:

1. *The underlying need for the drugs*. We echo some of the concerns of parents who wonder if the medical establishment is not "medicalizing" typical childhood misbehavior in some instances. Is it our children that need to be changed or our attitudes toward them? Should they be medicated because it's the easiest thing to do when no one has the time to look more deeply into the reasons for their behavior? Should a child be medicated because a teacher prefers a more compliant, conforming child, when the child might only be bored senseless in an unstimulating day care or classroom environment?

2. *The safety of the drugs*. Although Ritalin has been used for years and appears to have a good safety profile, it has known side effects, such as depression, lethargy, insomnia, lack of appetite, motor tics, moodiness, irritability, headaches, stomachaches, and slower growth. These side effects occur more often and are more severe in children under five than in their school-aged siblings. We are also concerned about its potential long-term effects on brain chemistry, especially now that it is being used so commonly in preschoolers, whose developing brains are very plastic and easily influenced. The stimulant drugs could theoretically affect brain development

and function, especially in the area of serotonin production. Unfortunately, children taking stimulants and other psychotropic drugs today are unknowingly participating in a large-scale drug-safety experiment.

3. *The misuse of the drugs*. Ritalin is often the first choice of treatment in even mild cases of ADD, despite recommendations that it be given to preschool children only in the most severe cases, and that it not be given before behavioral interventions have been tried. The diagnosis of ADD is often so subjective that ADD drugs are frequently prescribed to children who don't even have ADD. When a prescription stimulant is prescribed, the doctor should follow up with blood pressure checks every three months and regular behavioral follow-ups to adjust dosages and make sure there's a continued need for the medication. Beware of abuse by older children—in 2006, Ritalin was one of the three drugs most commonly abused by eighth graders.

An Integrative Program for ADD

Dr. D prescribes far fewer of the stimulant drugs than do most practices his size. That's because he combines a rigorous diagnostic process with strong support from parents in making nutritional, behavioral, environmental, and other changes to support their children's educational success. Dr. Russ typically sees patients who have already been given a diagnosis of ADD but whose parents are committed to finding complementary options, or even alternatives, to conventional medicines. He finds that some children clearly require pharmaceutical intervention, at least in the short term, while others do well with a multifaceted approach that aims to show a child he has more control over his situation than he thought. Some of these children successfully come off all medications, while others can be maintained on much lower doses than are usually employed.

An integrative approach should include the following steps:

1. *Having confidence in the diagnosis*. Make sure you, your child, her teachers, coaches, and others provide feedback to your child's doctor, so the doctor can get a true picture of your child's behavior and function. Insist on documentation of your child's observed functional impairment over a period of time. Consider any other medical conditions that could be causing difficulties at school. Take a frank look at any stresses in her life (and your own) or aspects of your parenting style or home environment that might be affecting her behavior.

2. *Holding off on medication unless clearly indicated.* We reserve the use of stimulant drugs for the more severe cases of ADD, as in our experience most other cases can be significantly improved without the use of prescription drugs. On rare occasions we initiate drug therapy as a bridge treatment until the best alternative for an individual child has been identified.

3. *Setting up consistent routines at home.* Children with ADD often improve dramatically in a calmer, more predictable environment. Consider filling out a home-and-school planner with your child to structure daily routines. Turn off the TV, limit fast-paced computer games, play soft music, set age-appropriate guidelines for behavior, and make mealtimes and bedtimes more relaxed and pleasant. Give your child time each day to blow off some steam through physical activity.

4. *Modifying the learning environment.* Extensive educational testing is an important part of the diagnostic process with ADD. An educational professional can identify coexistent learning disabilities and recommend specific learning behaviors or strategies that help kids with ADD stay on task and do better in school. Armed with a diagnosis, you may also be able to negotiate modifications in the classroom and obtain additional education support services that make it easier for your child to focus his thoughts and energy.

5. *Reinforcing desired behavior with praise and small rewards.*

6. *Teaching self-regulatory and relaxation skills.* Techniques such as EEG (brain wave) biofeedback, guided imagery, or clinical hypnosis can help children reduce anxiety, improve self-control, manage sleep problems, and change attitudes about school. A physical form of relaxation, such as yoga or walking meditation, may be even more appealing.

7. *Adding essential fatty acids to your child's diet*. Children with ADD, especially those who also have dry skin or eczema, appear to have lower blood levels of essential fatty acids, which are important constituents of brain cells. While not a cure, additional omega-3 fatty acids in the diet could have a positive impact. Make sure your child is getting an adequate amount of these fatty acids through foods such as cold-water fish, flaxseed meal, or through omega-3 supplements (4 to 6 grams a day for children over eight).

8. *Testing for food sensitivities*. Certain additives and foods appear to make ADD symptoms worse in a significant percentage of children. Try a three-week elimination diet that cuts out one problematic food at a time, such as wheat, corn, milk, preservatives, and food colorings like tartrazine (FD&C Yellow No. 5). A diet high in low-quality carbohydrates (white flour, white sugar, and fructose) may also be associated with behavioral problems, so provide a more nutrient-dense diet with some protein to balance the carbohydrates. Results of studies using special diets for ADD, like the Feingold Diet, are contradictory. We don't recommend such diets because the evidence for benefit isn't strong yet, and adhering to such a strict diet can be extremely stressful on caregivers, which could make symptoms worse in their children.

9. *Limiting exposure to environmental toxins*. (See chapter 8.)

Despite these helpful strategies, there is clearly a subset of kids—generally the most impulsive and hyperactive—who will need stimulant medications. Even if it is decided that your child does need prescription stimulants, these natural approaches may reduce the dosage of drug required and the duration that they are needed. Parents should make it clear to children with ADD that their difference is not a bad thing—that in fact they may be more creative or gifted in other ways than their classmates.

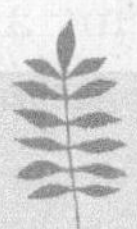

TIP: Don't forget to take care of yourself. A child with ADD can be quite a handful–lovable, but very, very stimulating. Take time to recharge your batteries so you can continue to deal with your child with love and patience.

CHAPTER 23

Sleep Issues

It would be wonderful if every child slept like a baby, but—unfortunately for their parents—many don't. In our fast-paced modern world, sleep is too often shorted by children and their parents. Yet sleep (or the lack of it) can have wide-ranging effects on the cardiovascular, endocrine, immune, and nervous systems.

While your children sleep, their bodies are resting and repairing, and their minds are processing the day's events and storing memories. Many hormones, including those responsible for appetite and growth, are secreted into the blood during sleep. When children don't get enough sleep, they suffer the effects. And it's not just that they get cranky. Inadequate sleep can contribute to fatigue, irritability, daytime drowsiness, difficulties concentrating, learning problems, increased risk of viral infection, depression, and even obesity.

How much sleep should your child get? Experts agree that kids in every age group are not getting the sleep they need. They recommend:

14 to 15 hours a day of sleep for infants three to eleven months
12 to 14 hours a day for kids one and two years of age
11 to 13 hours for kids three to six
10 to 11 hours for kids seven to eleven
8 ½ to 9 ½ hours for adolescents

more on . . .

PARENTS AND SLEEP

Kids aren't the only ones who need the rest and restoration of sleep. Good parents need enough sleep to stay sane too. Don't get caught in the endless cycle of waking up tired, grabbing a cup of coffee, then another and another throughout the day, and then being overcaffeinated and unable to sleep. Adequate sleep can reduce stress, improve performance (forget those all-nighters), increase patience, and even help new moms lose their "baby fat." If you can't get enough sleep at night, fit in a refreshing twenty-minute nap during the day.

Setting the Stage for Sleep

If your child has trouble falling or staying asleep at night, look first at what he does during the day. In his book *Healing Night*, psychologist Ruben Naiman says, "A good night's sleep is about a good day's waking." A day in which your child eats well, exercises, and manages stress successfully leads to a better night's sleep. Days filled with anxiety, caffeinated beverages, high-sugar foods, and exciting entertainment can make it hard to sleep at night. Here are some tips to help bring on the Sandman:

- *Establish bedtime rituals.* Create a routine around going to bed that provides relaxation and low stimulation—a warm bath, a warm drink, story time, prayers, quiet music, a guided imagery or relaxation tape. Give the child his favorite stuffed toy or blankie during the rituals so he associates them with comfort and rest.

- *Reduce media stimulation.* Turn off the TV/video/computer thirty minutes or more before bed, lower the lights, and quiet the house. Don't put a TV in a child's bedroom where it cannot be supervised, and don't let your kids go to bed with cell phone in hand.

- *Make the bedroom a good place to sleep.* Use curtains to block out light. Make sure the bed and pillows are comfortable and the room feels safe.

▶ *Unwind stress with a brief, relaxing massage.* A little lavender oil mixed into moisturizing cream adds a little herbal soporific.

▶ *Make sure the child gets some exercise during the day and some exposure to sunlight to normalize his or her sleep/wake patterns.*

▶ *Cut out caffeine.* Kids aged three to ten who drink at least one caffeinated beverage a day sleep about 35 minutes less a night, for a weekly sleep loss of over three hours. Watch out for high-sugar foods before bedtime too.

Dealing with the Sleep-Resistant Child

Some babies—and children—seem to resist sleep with every fiber of their being. If your baby over five months old wakes frequently in the night, it's probably time to move her to a room of her own. Infants are so tuned in to their mothers that just sensing or smelling their presence can wake them up. With a baby monitor in place, you'll be able to hear when she needs to be fed or changed.

If your baby over three months of age cries and cries when you put him down to sleep, try something that at first seems counterintuitive (if not unkind): Let him cry a little longer each night. When you do go to him, of course you can offer him the love and concern you always do, but simply wait a few minutes longer each night. Over the course of a week or two, he should finally settle down to sleep more easily.

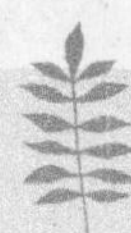

TIP: To help a child learn to associate bed—not you—with sleep, just rock or nurse her until she's drowsy, then put her in her bed to sleep. Don't put her to bed in her stroller or she'll still be sleeping there when she's a toddler.

What do you do with an older child who always drags out the bedtime process? If parents want to have any down time at all, they've got to get their kids on a regular bedtime schedule. We think you'll find that kids actually like a little routine in their lives. Turn off the media machines 30 to 60 minutes before bed and use that time for a bath, to read or be read to, or to listen to relaxing music. The kids should know that the lights go out at a certain time and that parents will not be making any visits after that. Sometimes the guilty parties here are not the kids but the parents, especially working parents who try to extend their treasured time with the kids. Just remember that kids need sleep as well as love.

Bed-Wetting

Bed-wetting (enuresis) is the inability of a toilet-trained child to hold urine throughout the night. It can be caused by physical problems such as obstructive sleep apnea, but generally it has an emotional basis. In fact, it's often tied to stress at home, especially the arrival of a newborn. Most bed-wetting is outgrown by age six, but the strategies below should speed its departure:

- *Don't wake a sleeping child to pee*. You want him to develop confidence in his own ability to wake up.

- *Maintain a positive attitude, and use positive language*. Congratulate her on "staying dry all night," not on "not wetting the bed."

- *Keep a chart with stars for dry nights*. Then give a little reward at the end for a positive reinforcement.

- *Try a guided imagery book or tape on staying dry*. Self-regulation hypnosis works very successfully in cooperative kids.

Parasomnias

The most common sleep disorders in children are parasomnias—nightmares, night terrors, and sleepwalking. A *nightmare* is a vivid and terrifying dream that wakes a child up abruptly and may make it hard to go back to sleep. They occur more frequently in creative kids, but decline in frequency with age. They are not worrisome, and children may simply be soothed and sent back to sleep.

Sleepwalking, or somnambulism, is an arousal disorder that occurs in deep sleep.

It will also be outgrown, so just make sure doors and windows are locked and the area is safe until then.

Night terrors is another arousal disorder occurring in deep sleep that is essentially harmless but a little scarier for parents to observe. A child with night terrors is agitated, confused, has large pupils, is sweating, is difficult to arouse, and may be screaming like a banshee. Try to gently calm the child by rocking or other form of soothing, keeping in mind that the child may not respond to soothing because he isn't really awake. Wait for the terror to end, then put him back to bed. He will usually fall quietly back to sleep and have no memory of the event the next day. If night terrors occur more often or become severe, take your child to the doctor to rule out unusual causes, like nocturnal seizures.

Snoring and Sleep-Disordered Breathing

Snoring in a child can have a number of causes from a cold or allergy to the more serious *sleep-disordered breathing* (SDB). SDB is the repeated partial or total collapse of upper airways, temporarily blocking airflow and stopping breathing. Kids are considered to have mild SDB if they snore at least three times a week and experience some sleep disturbances. The one in twenty kids with more severe SDB are considered to have obstructive sleep apnea.

The prevalence of sleep-disordered breathing is increasing as more and more children become overweight or obese. SDB shows up early in life and should be treated as early as possible to protect brain development and assure the child reaches his full intellectual potential. Other risk factors for SDB include oversized adenoids and tonsils (common in young children), craniofacial abnormalities, or chronic passive exposure to cigarette smoke.

Symptoms of SDB include hyperactivity, emotional ups and downs, attention problems, and difficulty completing tasks. Kids with SDB may be misdiagnosed as having ADHD, but when their breathing problem is relieved, the "ADHD" may disappear.

If you suspect your child has resistant sleep-disordered breathing, talk to his doctor about taking him to an ear, nose, and throat specialist for evaluation.

Sudden Infant Death Syndrome

Sudden infant death syndrome (SIDS, or crib death) is the leading cause of death in children under a year old. SIDS occurs suddenly and unpredictably, but you can reduce the risk of SIDS by doing the following:

- *Put your baby down to sleep on her back, not her belly*. This Back to Sleep campaign by the AAP has halved SIDS deaths in the United States. If your baby has GERD, discuss sleeping position with the doctor.
- *Refrain from smoking*. Babies whose mothers smoked while pregnant are three times more likely to die of SIDS; those who are passively exposed to cigarette smoke are twice as likely to die of SIDS.
- *Abstain from alcohol or other drugs*. Parents who drink or use drugs should never share the bed with an infant.
- *Making the crib safer*. Use a firm mattress, and no sheepskins, comforters, stuffed toys, or pillows in the crib.

ACKNOWLEDGMENTS

Stuart: First to my loving wife, Ruby, who supported and nurtured me every step of the way from concept through the writing of this book. It was your belief in the importance of finding better ways to care for kids that kept me moving forward. Without your patience and skill in caring for our children's needs I would not have been able to do this work. You are truly a master of stress management. The way you encourage healthy habits in our kids and keep me focused on the importance of family even as I strive to achieve professionally could provide a template for all families. Your insistence twenty years ago on the importance of our eating dinner together is just one proof of your vision as a mom and family leader. Thanks also to my mom and dad, Helen and Teddy Ditchek—of blessed memory—who instilled in me the inner light that allowed me to dream and to care for people with compassion and without bias. Their warmth continues to emanate from all those who knew them and loved them. I would like to thank Jane Friedman, who encouraged me to develop this book and opened my eyes to the privilege of educating the many rather than the few. It was Jane who introduced me to the important and groundbreaking works of Dr. Andrew Weil. Andy's warmth and loving logic have inspired me to a new level of compassionate care for my patients.

I have been most inspired professionally by memories of my own pediatrician as a child, Dr. Morris Steiner. This doctor's doctor was a leader in the field of general pediatrics and an expert in the treatment of the many children with tuberculosis in the 1950s. This model of a generalist, whose rich experiences eventually gave him expertise in specific areas, strongly influenced my practice philosophy and style—minimally invasive, maximally diagnostic, and always reassuring. His gentle way and openness with mothers in a generation when parents relied wholly on their pediatricians for knowledge became a model for me. I believe Dr. Steiner was truly one of the first integrative pediatricians in the United States.

I would like to thank my mentor, Laurence Finberg, M.D., whose meticulous guidance throughout my training years at SUNY–Downstate, Kings County Medical Center, was a critical basis for my future work. Steve Shelov, M.D., chairman of Pediatrics at Maimonides Medical Center, has been a great friend and teacher. His open-minded approach to pediatric care makes him a real leader in his field. Thanks to integrative dentist extraordinaire Robert Richter, D.D.S., another pioneer. A special thanks goes to Felicia Axelrod, M.D., and the entire Familial Dysautonomia Division at NYU, whose confidence helped me gain the expertise to care for these incredible families.

To my campers and the unique staff at Chai Lifeline Camp Simcha Special, I thank you for teaching me courage and the spiritual strength needed when faced with the challenges of serious illness. You are all my heroes and models for living a full and complete life. You have taught me that a healer must first be a friend.

Most important, I'd like to thank Russ Greenfield and Lynn Willeford for being such great friends and colleagues. Russ's unique career perspectives and warm insights and Lynn's keen writing, editorial skills, and understanding of the medical landscape made this book a robust reality. I consider you to be the closest of friends and look forward to many future endeavors together.

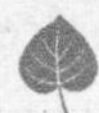

Russell: I must begin by recognizing the selfless devotion and support of my wife, Julia, who walks in beauty, and the stardust of our children, Abby and Jonathan. Your love makes anything possible, and everything beautiful. I count my blessings daily.

I reflect gratefully on my own childhood. I have my mom, Sophie; my dad, Alexander; and my brother, Michael, to thank for my growing up a whole child. They lovingly instilled in me a sense of family, the desire to learn, and a childlike appreciation for beauty and innocence. Individually and collectively, they are my role models for character, courage, and dignity. I also offer gratitude and love to Jean and Julius Greenfield, Betty and James Stanley, and all the rest of my family.

I am grateful to my teacher and friend, Andrew Weil, M.D., who dreams of a better world and—not satisfied just to dream—works to make it so. I owe a debt of gratitude to Tracy Gaudet, M.D., who supported my journey and enriched my life at great personal sacrifice. I thank my partners in the first class of the Program in Integrative Medicine at the University of Arizona Health Sciences Center for their support and camaraderie during our unique time together: Wendy Kohatsu, M.D.; Roberta Lee, M.D.; and Karen Koffler, M.D. Thank you to everyone at the Program in Integrative Medicine, who gave freely that I might learn, and to the faculty of the Department of Emergency Medicine at Harbor–UCLA Medical Center, for taking a wide-eyed boy and turning him into a doctor, and for instilling in me the love of teaching. To my friends at Carolinas Integrative Health, thank you for your love and partnership, and for warm memories of the magical time that we shared together as one. I humbly thank all the people whom I've cared for as patients, who allowed me to witness their journeys and have taught me so much about myself and about life.

To my friends, especially Keith Nelson and Colleen Grochowski, thank you for your enthusiastic belief in me.

A chance encounter in a gift shop led to the realization of shared dreams and this book. My coauthors, Stuart Ditchek, M.D., and Lynn Willeford, are exceptionally kind human beings, gifted artists, and compassionate healers (even though Lynn has no initials after her name). The fact that we came together is evidence of there being order in this world, and I am grateful beyond measure for the time we have spent together.

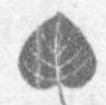

Lynn: I want to thank my husband, Blake; my son, Brook; my mother, Audrey Baston; my sister, Laurie Watts; my dad, Les Baston; and my daughter-in-love, Wendi, for their unwavering belief in my abilities and their steadfast love. I could ask for no fiercer advocates (and no better tech support). I am also grateful to my South Whidbey support team; to Andy Weil, who opened my eyes all those years ago to a more expansive vision of health; to the writers and editors at *Dr. Andrew Weil's Self Healing*; and, of course, to my bright, compassionate, skilled, and funny docs, Russ and Stu.

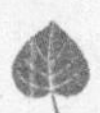

We would all like to thank Andrew Weil, M.D., for his foreword; the late Michael Rothenberg, M.D., and Jo Rothenberg for their thoughts on our original outline; and Steven Shelov, M.D., for his invaluable input along the way. We want to take this opportunity to honor Andrew Weil, who through force of intellect, a belief in the indomitable human spirit, and the desire to do good in the world, is helping redefine the practice of medicine.

We would also like to thank the following generous people for their information and feedback on specific chapters: Cyndi Thomson Ph.D., R.D.; Bob Lutz, M.D., and his wife Amy Lutz, M.Ed.; Ken Bromberg, M.D.; Susan Schacter, M.S., R.D.; Rosa Schnyer, L.Ac.; Steve Gurgevich, Ph.D.; Francis Brinker, N.D.; Herbert Needleman, M.D.; Judyth Reichenberg-Ullman, N.D.; Ceci McCarten, M.D.; Larry Sugarman, M.D.; John Mark, M.D.; Sharon McDonough-Means, M.D.; Michael O'Connell, M.D.; Ilene M. Spector, D.O.; Margaret Avery-Moon, N.C.T.M.B.; Andrea Morken; and Susan Ferguson, R.N., B.S.N., R.Y.T.

We are grateful to Jane Friedman for the chance to revise and publish again a book that was years ahead of its time when it first came out in 2001, and to our editor Mary Ellen O'Neill for making the process such a pleasant one. Thanks to all the wonderful folks at Collins Living for their support, talent, and continual good cheer, especially Matthew Patin, Lelia Mander, Kimberly Chocolaad, and April Sirianni. Thanks to Jaime Putorti, Amanda Kain, and Alexis Seabrook for making the book look both graceful and accessible. And finally, we thank our agent Richard Pine for the guidance he has offered to a couple of upstart doctor-authors.

Last, we offer thanks to the true leaders of integrative medicine, those who forged paths alone, believing not only in the medicine of the known but also in the medicine of the possible.

We dedicate this book to parents and children around the world.

RESOURCES

Here are some of our favorite books, newsletters, CDs, DVDs, organizations, Web sites, and other sources of additional information on the topics covered in this book. Web sites come and go, so take the Internet addresses listed here with a grain of salt, and be prepared to use a search engine to locate an organization's new site.

General Information on Integrative Medicine

Eight Weeks to Optimum Health, Andrew Weil, M.D. (Knopf, 1997)

Integrative Medicine: An Introduction to the Art and Science of Healing, audiotape/CD, Andrew Weil, M.D. (Sounds True, 2001)

Natural Health, Natural Medicine: The Complete Guide to Wellness and Self-Care for Optimum Health, Andrew Weil, M.D. (Houghton Mifflin, 2004)

The Best Alternative Medicine: What Works? What Does Not? Kenneth Pelletier, M.D. (Simon & Schuster, 2007)

The Mayo Clinic Book of Alternative Medicine: The New Approach to Using the Best of Natural Therapies and Conventional Medicine, The Mayo Clinic (Time, 2007)

Dr. Andrew Weil's Self Healing newsletter, (800) 523-3296; www.drweilselfhealing.com

Dr. Andrew Weil's Web site, www.drweil.com

National Center for Complementary and Alternative Medicine of the National Institutes of Health, (888) 644-6226; www.nccam.nih.gov/

University of Arizona Program in Integrative Medicine, www.integrativemedicine.arizona.edu

General Information on Pediatrics

Caring for Your Baby and Young Child: Birth to Age 5, American Academy of Pediatrics, Steven Shelov, M.D., editor (Bantam, 2004)

Caring for Your School-Age Child: Ages 5 to 12, American Academy of Pediatrics, Edward Schur, M.D., editor (Bantam, 1999)

Everyday Blessings: The Inner Work of Mindful Parenting, Myla Kabat-Zinn and Jon Kabat-Zinn (Hyperion, 1998)

The Doctors' Book of Home Remedies, Debora Tkac, editor (Rodale, 2003)

The Natural Nursery: The Parent's Guide to Ecologically Sound, Non-Toxic, Safe, and Healthy Baby Care, Louis Pottkotter, M.D. (Contemporary Books, 1994)

What to Expect When You're Expecting (2002), *What to Expect the First Year* (2004), and *What to Expect the Toddler Years* (1996), Arlene Eisenberg, Heidi Murkoff, and Sandra Hathaway, B.S.N. (Workman)

Dr. Ditchek's Web site, www.drditchek.com

American Academy of Family Physicians, www.familydoctor.org

American Academy of Pediatrics, www.aap.org/parents.html

PubMed, the National Institutes of Health research database, www.ncbi.nlm.nih/gov/PubMed/

The Nemours Center for Children's Health, www.kidshealth.org

Immunity

Health and Healing: The Philosophy of Integrative Medicine and Optimum Health, Andrew Weil, M.D. (Houghton Mifflin, 2004)

Molecules of Emotion: The Science Behind Mind/Body Medicine, Candace Pert, Ph.D. (Simon & Schuster 1999)

How Your Immune System Works, www.howstuffworks.com/immune-system.htm

Vaccinations

Vaccinated: One Man's Quest to Defeat the World's Deadliest Diseases, Paul Offit, M.D. (HarperCollins, 2007)

Vaccinating Your Child: Questions and Answers for the Concerned Parent, Sharon Humiston, M.D., and Cynthia Good (Peachtree, 2003)

For more on the vaccine and autism controversy, see www.briandeer.com/mmr/lancet-summary.htm

Immunization Action Coalition, www.immunize.org

National Immunization Program, www.cdc.gov/vaccines/

Antibiotics

Breaking the Antibiotic Habit: A Parent's Guide to Coughs, Colds, Ear Infections, and Sore Throats, Paul Offit, M.D., and Louis Bell, M.D. (John Wiley, 1999)

The Antibiotic Paradox: How Miracle Drugs Are Destroying the Miracle, Stuart Levy, M.D. (HarperCollins, 2002)

Alliance for the Prudent Use of Antibiotics, www.tufts.edu/med/apua/

Fact sheets from the National Institute of Allergies and Infectious Diseases, www.niaid.nih.gov/topics/AntimicrobialResistance.htm

National Center for Infectious Disease, www.cdc.gov/drugresistance/community/

Nutrition

Breastfeeding Your Baby, Sheila Kitzinger (Knopf, 1998)

Child of Mine: Feeding with Love and Good Sense, Ellyn Satter (Bull Publishing, 2000)

Deceptively Delicious: Simple Secrets to Get Your Kids Eating Good Food, Jessica Seinfeld (HarperCollins, 2007)

Eating Well for Optimum Health: The Essential Guide to Food, Diet, and Nutrition, Andrew Weil, M.D. (Knopf, 2000)

Feeding Your Child for Lifelong Health, Susan B. Roberts, Ph.D., and Melvin B. Heyman, M.D., with Lisa Tracy (Bantam, 1999)

Food Politics, Marion Nestle, Ph.D. (University of California Press, 2007)

How to Get Your Child to Eat . . . But Not Too Much, Ellyn Satter (Bull Publishing, 1987)

The Crazy Makers: How the Food Industry Is Destroying Our Minds and Harming Our Children, Carol Simontacchi (Jeremy Tarcher, 2007)

The Mash and Smash Cookbook: Fun and Yummy Recipes Every Kid Can Make! Marion Buck-Murray (John Wiley, 1997)

The Nursing Mother's Companion, Kathleen Huggins (Harvard Common Press, 2005)

The Sneaky Chef: Simple Strategies for Hiding Healthy Foods in Kids' Favorite Meals, Missy Chase Lapine (Running Press, 2007)

The Yale Guide to Children's Nutrition, William Tamborlane, M.D., editor (Yale University Press, 1997)

What To Eat, Marion Nestle, Ph.D. (North Point, 2007)

Dr. Russ at the Harris Teeter nutrition site, www.harristeeter.com/yourwellness/yourwellness_for_life/yourwellness_for_life.aspx

BAM! interactive health Web site for kids nine to thirteen, www.bam.gov

Best fish Web site, www.oceansalive.org/eat.cfm

Farmers' Market Nutrition Program, www.fns.usda.gov/wic/

Farmers' markets are listed at www.ams.usda.gov/farmersmarkets

Food and Drug Administration Center for Food Safety and Applied Nutrition, (800) 332-4010; www.foodsafety.gov

Lifecycle Nutrition at the USDA Food and Nutrition Information Center, www.fnic.nal.usda.gov

National Farm to School Program, www.farmtoschool.org

Nutrition Action, newsletter of the Center for Science in the Public Interest, www.cspinet.org

Nutrition and Your Child newsletter and other materials at USDA Children's Nutrition Research Center at Baylor College of Medicine, www.kidsnutrition.org

Physical Fitness/Obesity

Dynamic Physical Education for Elementary School Children, R. P. Pangrazi (Allyn and Bacon, 1998)

Promoting Physical Activity: A Guide for Community Action (Centers for Disease Control, 1999)

Your Child's Fitness: Practical Advice for Parents, Susan Kalish, for the American Running and Fitness Association (Human Kinetics, 1996)

Alliance for a Healthier Generation, www.healthiergeneration.org

American Association for the Child's Right to Play, www.ipausa.org

BMI for children, www.cdc.gov/nccdphp/dnpa/bmi/childrens_bmi/about_childrens_bmi.htm

Stress Management

Breathing, the Master Key to Self Healing, cassette/CD, Andrew Weil, M.D. (Sounds True, 1999)

Conscious Breathing: Breathwork for Health, Stress Release, and Personal Mastery, Gay Hendricks, Ph.D. (Bantam, 1995)

Cool Cats, Calm Kids: Relaxation and Stress Management for Young People, Mary L. Williams (Impact, 1996)

Full Catastrophe Living: Using the Wisdom of the Body and Mind to Face Stress, Pain, and Illness, Jon Kabat-Zinn (Piatkus, 2001)

Relax, Catherine O'Neill Grace (Child's Play, 1993)

Seven Times the Sun: Guiding Your Child Through the Rhythms of the Day, Shea Darian (Gilead, 1999)

Stress-Proofing Your Child: Mind-Body Exercises to Enhance Your Child's Health, Sheldon Lewis and Sheila Kay Lewis (Bantam, 1996)

The Wellness Book: The Comprehensive Guide to Maintaining Health and Treating Stress-Related Illness, Herbert Benson, M.D., and Eileen Stuart, R.N., M.S. (Fireside, 1993)

Environmental Issues

Home Safe Home: Protecting Yourself and Your Family from Everyday Toxics and Harmful Household Products, Debra Lynn Dadd (Jeremy Tarcher, 1997)

Last Child in the Woods: Saving Our Children from Nature-Deficit Disorder, Richard Luov (Algonquin, 2006)

Raising Baby Green: The Earth-Friendly Guide to Pregnancy, Childbirth, and Baby Care, Alan Greene, M.D., et al. (Jossey-Bass, 2007)

Raising Healthy Children in a Toxic World: 101 Smart Solutions for Every Family, Herbert Needleman, M.D., and Philip Landrigan, M.D. (Rodale, 2002)

The Geography of Childhood: Why Children Need Wild Places, Gary Paul Nabhan and Stephen Trimble (Beacon, 1995)

Books for Young People on Environmental Issues (grades K–6 and 7–12), www.epa.state.il.us/kids/teachers/books.html

Children's Environmental Health Network, www.cehn.org

Drinking Water Hotline, (800) 426-4791; www.epa.gov/safewater/

Environmental Concepts Made Easy, http://e.hormone.tulane.edu

Environmental Working Group, www.ewg.org

EPA Lead Web site, www.epa.gov/lead or (800) 424-LEAD

National Geographic's Green Guide, www.thegreenguide.com

Natural Resources Defense Council Green Living, www.nrdc.org/greenliving/

Office of Children's Health Protection (EPA), www.yosemite.epa.gov/ochp/ochpweb.nsf/content/whatwe.htm

Safe Kids USA, www.usa-safekids.org

Cultural Issues

Put Your Heart on Paper: Staying Connected in a Loose-Ends World, Henriette Anne Klauser (Bantam, 1995)

Raising Children in a Socially Toxic Environment, James Garbarino (Jossey-Bass, 1999)

Entertainment Software Rating Board, www.esrb.org

Movie ratings, www.filmratings.com

National Institute on Media and the Family, www.mediafamily.org

Mind/Body Medicine

Anatomy of an Illness as Perceived by the Patient, Norman Cousins (Norton, 2005)

Be the Boss of Your Body, books on sleep, pain, and stress, Timothy Culbert, M.D., and Rebecca Kajander, CPNP (Free Spirit, 2007)

Earthlight: New Meditations for Children, Maureen Garth (HarperOne, 1997)

Guided Imagery for Self-Healing, Martin Rossman, M.D. (H. J. Kramer, 2000)

Healing and the Mind, Bill Moyers (Main Street Books, 1995)
Meditating with Children: The Art of Concentration and Centering, Deborah Rozman (Integral Yoga, 2002)
Moonbeam: A Book of Meditations for Children, Maureen Garth (HarperOne, 1999)
The Relaxation Response, Herbert Benson, M.D., with Miriam Klipper (Harper, 2000)
Timeless Healing: The Power and Biology of Belief, Herbert Benson, M.D., with Marg Stark (Scribner, 1997)
YogaKids, DVD, Marsha Wenig (Living Arts, 2004)
YogaKids: Educating the Whole Child Through Yoga, Marsha Wenig (Stewart, Tabori, and Chang, 2003)
Academy for Guided Imagery, academyforguidedimagery.com
American Music Therapy Association, www.musictherapy.org
American Society of Clinical Hypnosis, www.asch.net/genpubinfo.htm
Biofeedback Certification Institute of America, bcia.org
Guided Imagery Resource Center, www.healthjourneys.com
Health Journeys imagery resources, www.healthjourneys.com
Tranceformation hypnosis resources, www.tranceformation.com

Manual Medicine

Acupressure's Potent Points: A Guide to Self-Care for Common Ailments, Michael Reed Gach (Bantam, 1990)
Discovering the Body's Wisdom, Mirka Knaster (Bantam, 1996)
American Massage Therapy Association, www.amtamassage.org
American Osteopathic Association, (800) 621-1773; www.osteopathic.org
The Cranial Academy, www.cranialacademy.org

Botanical Medicine

Herbal Prescriptions for Health and Healing, Donald Brown, N.D. (Lotus, 2003)
The Encyclopedia of Natural Medicine, Michael Murray, N.D., and Joseph Pizzorno, N.D. (Three Rivers Press, 1997)

The Healing Power of Herbs, Michael Murray, N.D. (Gramercy, 2004)
Alternative Medicine at Rx List, the Internet Drug Index, www.rxlist.com
American Botanical Council, www.herbalgram.org
HerbMed of the Alternative Medicine Foundation, www.herbmed.org

Alternative Systems of Medicine

Traditional Chinese Medicine

Between Heaven and Earth: A Guide to Chinese Medicine, Harriet Beinfield Lac and Efrem Korngold Lac, O.M.D. (Ballantine, 1991)
Encounters with Qi: Exploring Chinese Medicine, David Eisenberg, M.D., and Thomas Lee Wright (W. W. Norton, 1995)
The Web That Has No Weaver: Understanding Chinese Medicine, Ted Kaptchuk, O.M.D. (McGraw-Hill, 2000)
American Academy of Medical Acupuncture, www.medicalacupuncture.org
American Association of Oriental Medicine, www.aaaomonline.org
National Certification Commission for Acupuncture and Oriental Medicine, www.nccaom.org

Homeopathic Medicine

Healing with Homeopathy, Wayne Jonas, M.D., and Jennifer Jacobs, M.D. (Grand Central, 1998)
Homeopathic Medicine for Children and Infants, Dana Ullmann (Tarcher, 1992)
Homeopathic Self-Care: The Quick and Easy Guide for the Whole Family, Robert Ullman, N.D., and Judyth Reichenberg-Ullman, N.D. (Three Rivers Press, 1997)
Homeopathic Education Services, www.homeopathic.com
National Center for Homeopathy, www.homeopathic.org

Energy Medicine

Accepting Your Power to Heal: Personal Practice Therapeutic Touch, Dolores Kreiger, Ph.D., R.N. (Bear and Company, 1993)

Healing Words, Larry Dossey, M.D. (HarperOne, 1997)

How People Heal: Exploring the Scientific Basis of Subtle Energy in Healing, Diane Goldner (Hampton Roads, 2003)

Prayer Is Good Medicine, Larry Dossey, M.D. (HarperOne, 1997)

Reiki: A Comprehensive Guide, Pamela Miles (Tarcher, 2006)

The Living Energy Universe: A Fundamental Discovery that Transforms Science and Medicine, Gary Schwartz, Ph.D., and Linda Russek, Ph.D. (Hampton Roads, 2006)

The Spiritual Life of Children, Robert Coles (Mariner, 1991)

The Touch of Healing: Energizing the Body, Mind, and Spirit with Jin Shin Jyutsu, Alice Burmeister and Tom Monte (Bantam, 1997)

An Introduction to Reiki, http://nccam.nih.gov/health/reiki/

Healing Touch International, www.healingtouchinternational.org

Allergy and Asthma

Chicken Soup for the Soul Healthy Living Series: Asthma, Norman Edelman, M.D., Jack Canning, and Mark Victor Hansen (HCI, 2006)

What Your Doctor May Not Tell You About Children's Allergies and Asthma, Paul Ehrlich, M.D., and Larry Chiaramonte, M.D. (Warner Books, 2003)

Allergy and Asthma Network—Mothers of Asthmatics, (800) 878-4403; www.aanma.org

American College of Allergy, Asthma, and Immunology, www.acaai.org

American Lung Association, (800) LUNGUSA; www.lungusa.org

Healthy Schools Network, www.healthyschools.org

National Jewish Research Center (specialists in respiratory illness), www.njc.org

The Food Allergy & Anaphylaxis Network, (800) 929-4040; www.foodallergy.org

Tummy Troubles

Breaking the Vicious Cycle: Intestinal Health Through Diet, Elaine Gottschall (Kirkton Press, 1994)

Attention Disorders

ADD/ADHD Behavior-Change Resource Kit , Grad Flick, Ph.D. (The Center for Applied Research in Education, 1998)

Please Don't Label My Child: Break the Doctor-Diagnosis-Drug Cycle and Discover Safe, Effective Choices for Your Child's Emotional Health, Scott Shannon, M.D., and Emily Heckman (Rodale, 2007)

Power Parenting for Children with ADD/ADHD: A Practical Parent's Guide for Managing Difficult Behavior, Grad Flick, Ph.D. (The Center for Applied Research in Education, 1996)

Ritalin-Free Kids, Judyth Reichenberg-Ullman, N.D., M.S.W., and Robert Ullman, N.D. (Three Rivers Press, 2000)

Sleep

Be the Boss of Your Sleep, Timothy Culbert, M.D., and Rebecca Kajander, CPNP (Free Spirit, 2007)

Healing Night: The Science and Spirit of Sleeping, Dreaming, and Awakening, Ruben Naiman, Ph.D. (Syren Books, 2006)

Healthy Sleep, CD, Andrew Weil, M.D., and Ruben Naiman, Ph.D. (Sounds True, 2007)

INDEX

5/13 ~~0~~ (7/12)
12/14 (3) 6/14
10/15 (4) 2/15